Wakefield Press

The Heaslip Bequest for Health

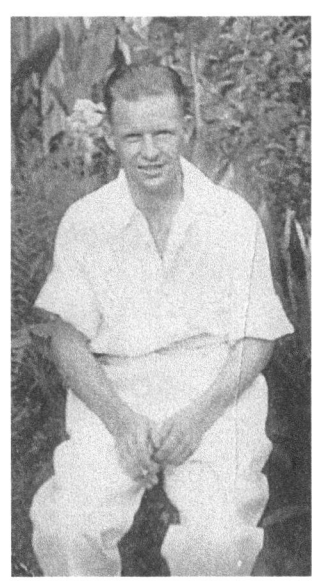

William Gordon Heaslip

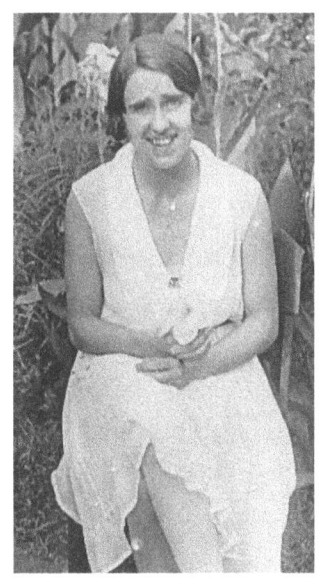

Barbara Kate Heaslip

Emeritus Professor **Peter McDonald** was the inaugural head of Microbiology and Infectious Diseases at Flinders University. In that role he joined the team that initiated the Flinders Medical Curriculum and established clinical and laboratory services for infectious diseases at Flinders Medical Centre.

From Flinders, his research into antibiotic dosing was applied internationally to reduce the rate of sepsis after surgery and employed in developing new antibiotics.

As Chair of the Commonwealth AIDS Research Grants committee, he coordinated research in Australia that underpinned the control of HIV in Australia and contributed to global control.

Professor McDonald played a role is health system reform by leading South Australian trials in coordinating health care and developing national infection-control guidelines.

He was awarded AM for services to Infectious Diseases and control of HIV/AIDS.

Robert Fitzsimons [PhD] has a special interest in South Australian history – one of several fields of historical research in which he was engaged over many years at Flinders University.

Peter Preece is the grandson of W.G. (Gordon) Heaslip, who provided access to the Heaslip Diaries and facilitated contact with Gordon's family.

The Heaslip Bequest for Health

Peter McDonald

with assistance from
Robert Fitzsimons and **Peter Preece**

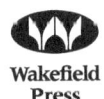

Wakefield
Press

Wakefield Press
16 Rose Street
Mile End
South Australia 5031
www.wakefieldpress.com.au

First published 2025

Copyright © Peter McDonald, 2025

All rights reserved. This book is copyright. Apart from any fair dealing for the purposes of private study, research, criticism or review, as permitted under the Copyright Act, no part may be reproduced without written permission. Enquiries should be addressed to the publisher.

Edited by Julia Beaven, Wakefield Press
Text designed and typeset by Jesse Pollard, Wakefield Press

ISBN 978 1 92338 815 4

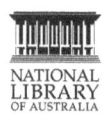 A catalogue record for this book is available from the National Library of Australia

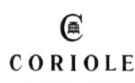 Wakefield Press thanks Coriole Vineyards for continued support

Contents

Preface — *vii*

Chapter 1
A Pioneering Family:
Gordon Heaslip's Heritage — 1

Chapter 2
Pathway to the Missions — 13

Chapter 3
Tropical Training, Papua — 24

Chapter 4
Research Career, South Australia — 49

Chapter 5
Queensland and World War II — 57

Chapter 6
Farming, Family, National Health — 70

Chapter 7
Gordon's Last Years:
Agriculture and a Bequest — 79

Chapter 8
Heaslip Bequest and
Flinders School of Medicine — 90

Appendix
National Health
by W.G. Heaslip — 110

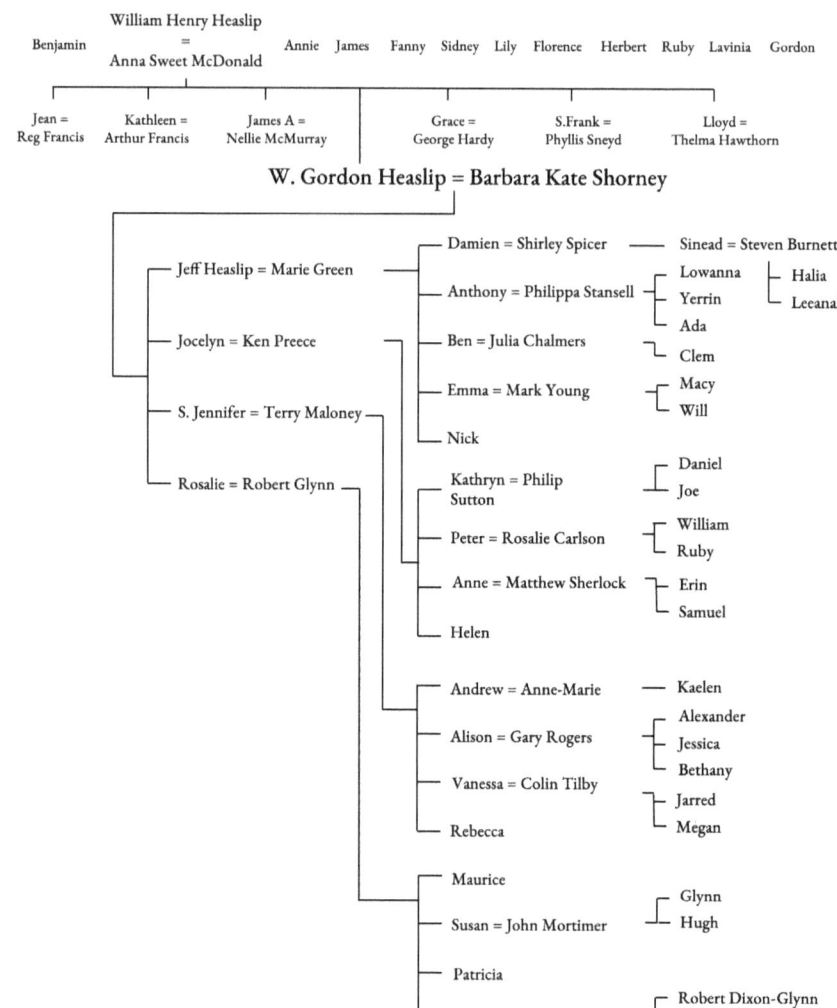

Preface

In 1985 I attended a meeting at the Executor Trustee and Agency Company of South Australia on behalf of the Dean of Flinders University School of Medicine. This meeting was convened to inform about a bequest by Wiliam Gordon Heaslip (known as Gordon) to improve medical education in South Australia.

Gordon Heaslip died in 1961 aged 59; the bequest became available after the death of his wife Barbara in 1982. The bequest specified that the executors establish a trust fund to be allocated to *a* medical school in South Australia whose teachers would guide students toward practising preventive as well as curative medicine. The executors received submissions from Adelaide and Flinders universities and chose to allocate the bequest to Flinders University. The university received the funds in 1986 and allocated them to the purposes specified in the bequest.

At the conclusion of the meeting of (mostly) lawyers, I asked who Gordon Heaslip was, and why he would have made such a bequest. The only information provided was a death certificate that indicated his cause of death as leukemia complicating polycythemia vera, and his occupation as a pathologist. Since I was a specialist pathologist and physician, I reckoned that I should have known about this benefactor, and I decided there must be a story behind this bequest.

By 2014, and now in retirement, I was able to spend time with Gordon Heaslip's family who were eager to share information about the Heaslip family and tell Gordon's story.

This book outlines the life and times of Gordon Heaslip, the rationale for his bequest, and its impact on medical teaching and health system reform. It is based in part on the Heaslip Diaries that were maintained by the head of clan and described events from 1851 to 1958. The private papers of the Heaslips are held in the Special Collections of Flinders University Library. Further information was provided by Gordon's daughter, Jocelyn Preece (née Heaslip) who wrote about her mother in *Adelaide Woman* (Victoria, 2007).

In writing this book I have been assisted by Dr Robert Fitzsimons, historian at Flinders University, Jocelyn Preece, and Gordon's grandson Peter Preece who provided access to the Heaslip Family Diaries.

When the bequest was awarded to Flinders University, I was a member of the team that developed the innovative Flinders Medical teaching program in the Flinders Medical Centre. The Heaslip Bequest assisted in developing that program.

Subsequently, I have participated in health system developments nationally to improve health outcomes in surgical sepsis, HIV/AIDS, and government strategies to improve national health through coordinated care.

In recent years, the Australian Government has initiated programs to improve health for all Australians through more effective primary health care and improved payment systems.

These objectives for Australia's future health align with Gordon Heaslip's aspirations for future health and the purposes of the Heaslip Bequest Trust Fund.

The opportunity presents for Flinders University to utilize the Heaslip Bequest to teach future doctors and health-care workers to achieve best health outcomes for the community.

Peter McDonald AM
Emeritus Professor Flinders University

Chapter 1

A Pioneering Family: Gordon Heaslip's Heritage

This is the story of William Gordon Heaslip. He was born in 1902 at Belton, in South Australia's Mid North, above the Goyder Line – harsh country, where rainfall was unreliable. His forebears had settled in this region some 50 years previously. They were in effect 'refugees' from the Great Irish Famine. Emigrants from County Cavan in the old province of Ulster, where for generations his folk had been farmers, Benjamin Heaslip and his family arrived at Port Adelaide on MV *Osceola* on the 6th of April, 1851. Great challenges lay before them. They worked hard, planned imaginatively, and evinced much stoicism, eventually prospering in this strange new land.

Such was Gordon Heaslip's background. After a colourful life he made a substantial bequest with a view to improving the health of South Australians. The family history and background that led to this bequest is outlined below.

From Ireland to Carrieton in South Australia
In 1845, famine was upon Ireland. Further devastation arose from cholera in the harsh winter of 1847. The Parish of Denn was in County Cavan, in the province of Ulster, one of the most severely affected counties (J. Crowley et al., *Atlas of the Great Irish Famine*, 2012).

In 1845, Benjamin Heaslip was a subsistence farmer in Balleyjamesduff on a mixed farm supporting a young family. Failed crops and pestilence were a burden on health and welfare, leading to malnutrition, persistent illness and premature deaths. Ben lost his beloved first wife Eliza Evans when their youngest child was six months old, leaving Benjamin with three children. He then married his second wife, Frances, with whom he had five more children.

Increasingly attracted by stories from the 'new world', Benjamin chose to relocate his family to Australia in 1850. County Cavan offered little more than continuing famine and pestilence, and migration seemed to be an attractive, if not the only, opportunity to support his family.

Somewhat like a package deal, the South Australian Company offered land in South Australia that could be selected in Britain, together with sea passage to South Australia. When the Heaslip family arrived in South Australia, the price of land was set at £1 per acre.

Heaslip arrival

Passage to South Australia was arranged for Ben, Frances and their eight children. On Christmas Eve 1850, Ben and his family departed Britain on the MV *Osceola* under the command of Captain Waite. While on the voyage to Australia Frances gave birth to another son. When the *Osceola* arrived at Port Adelaide on 6 April 1851, Ben, Frances and nine children disembarked.

Ben took his family to the Gawler River District, about 35 kilometres from Adelaide. There he procured land in the form of land grants. On 24 July 1852 he purchased Sections 3884 and 3891 and on October 11 Section 3889, all at £1 per acre. In October 1853 he paid £2/10/- per acre for eight acres adjacent to 3884. He accrued more sections over the years by mortgaging his original purchases and entering into lease agreements.

By 1853 a cottage had been built on the original holdings and 50 per cent of the land was under cultivation. In 1857 it was fully cultivated.

Ben and Frances with their children were the hard-working farmers sought by the South Australian Company. Ben's son, also named Ben, held a slaughtering licence and was reputedly responsible for preparing much of the meat consumed in the district. Ben senior purchased substantial tracts of land at £1 per acre and placed them in the name of Ben junior, who had just turned 21. He married Catherine Stafford and settled on his land, going on to raise a family of nine.

The quality of wheat produced in the lower north of South Australia fetched exceedingly high prices in Sydney and London. This enabled early settlers like the Heaslip family to embark on further land acquisitions by venturing capital on the expectation of producing high value crops and livestock.

Then tragedy struck. After just seven years in Australia Ben senior was riding home at dusk from a council meeting when he struck a tree branch, was thrown off his horse and was found dead by a neighbour. Ben was buried in the Smithfield Cemetery, Argent Lane, just north of Womma Road in Gawler. He left a widow and ten children, six of whom were minors.

Unsurprisingly at his age, Ben died intestate. The management of Ben's estate was complicated by the fact that it was necessary to establish Ben junior's relationship to his father and the fact that Frances was his stepmother. Documents were obtained from Ireland – copies of the first marriage to Ben senior, copies of the baptism of Benjamin junior, and a statement from Peter McEvoy of Peachy Belt, Ireland, wherein he stated that he had known Ben and Frances in Ireland before their marriage.

Ben senior's estate was not settled until 7 June 1858. Almost all of Benjamin senior's land was under a series of mortgages that were managed by executors of the estate – his sons Benjamin and James, and James Jones, a local farmer from Angle Vale who had financial dealings with the Heaslip family.

Frances released her right to dower on condition of receiving an annuity of £40 per annum until the younger boys came of age, when it would rise to £80. The annuity was legally recoverable from the income of some sections of her late husband's farms.

This diary excerpt illustrates how the Heaslip clan expanded their land holdings, taking every opportunity to purchase prime grain and grazing properties.

> *Benjamin 2nd received no land from the estate, he already owned the eastern property which had presumably been paid for by his*

father. The trustees were responsible for administering the estate, but James was appointed manager. Income was to go firstly toward the support of the younger children, after which James was entitled to £50 per annum as a management fee until the property was free from debt. In addition, he was entitled to one-third of the clear profits of the estate for a period of six years.

Each of Ben's daughters were to receive money, Lavinia who already married James Lindsay was to receive £150 within twelve months. Mary Ann, then aged 24, was to receive £200 plus 7.5% interest in April 1861. Ann, Elizabeth and Fanny were each to receive £200 on reaching 21 or on marrying with the consent of the trustees.

Each of Ben's other sons were to receive land. James was to be given the three sections near Undalya. He had already purchased in December 1857 Section 191, which was adjacent to his father's land, so he gained a compact property in a rich area of the state.

Frank (Francis) was to receive Section 3006 in the name of his mother Frances in 1863 when he reached 25 years of age. We do not know why he had to wait so long for his inheritance. He married Sophia Parker in 1863, and the land was transferred to him in April 1864. In May he sold it to John Williams allowing him a mortgage of £755 until Williams could find another mortgagee, which he did in February 1865. Meanwhile Frank had purchased land in the Hundred of Upper Wakefield near Auburn and had moved in there with his wife Sophia and their new-born son Benjamin Frances Aithcheson Heaslip.

The Heaslip Diaries recount notable family and commercial activities from the time of arrival in 1851. From 1872 James recorded land transactions, agricultural outputs (wheat, wool, stock), prices, machinery acquisitions, building works and important seasonal conditions. Importantly, these diaries are a record of family events. An introduction was written from available papers to describe family events from 1852, and James then continued with regular entries. The diaries were kept by the head of the extended family. James Heaslip authored the diaries until 1893, William Henry Heaslip from 1894–1934, and James Alexander Heaslip maintained the diaries until 1958.

The Heaslip holdings expanded from Gawler River through to Carrieton–Orroroo area and consolidated in Appila on an estate called Willow Park, which became the focus of family properties that ranged from Gilles Downs sheep station out from Iron Knob to grazing properties in the Tintinara district. However, Appila and Willow Park were the largest and most productive holdings from which the Heaslip estates developed.

From the time of settlement, the Heaslips were industrious and demonstrated care and understanding of farming based on generations of working small allotments in Ireland which allowed only subsistence living. The initial holdings in the Gawler area were quite small, but the opportunities of acquiring more land were taken up with alacrity by working together as an extended family. The prices received for wheat, wool and livestock were significantly more than mortgage costs, so in the early days of colonisation, quite large holdings were amassed.

Progressively, the family purchased more farming land to the north. Over the years they came to understand the vicissitudes of farming on the edge of a desert.

The landscape and history

The Mid North of South Australia contains great scenic beauty, prime agricultural land, and desert. Stark mountain ranges and undulating pastures interspersed with majestic eucalypts in mostly dry creeks and wide panoramas characterise this diverse region.

The country around Orroroo and Carrieton where the Heaslips established their first major holdings in 1855–60 was bounteous, but five years later drought set in: crops failed, animals had no feed, and many stations were abandoned. This boom-and-bust cycle became apparent by 1865, and Surveyor-General George Goyder was

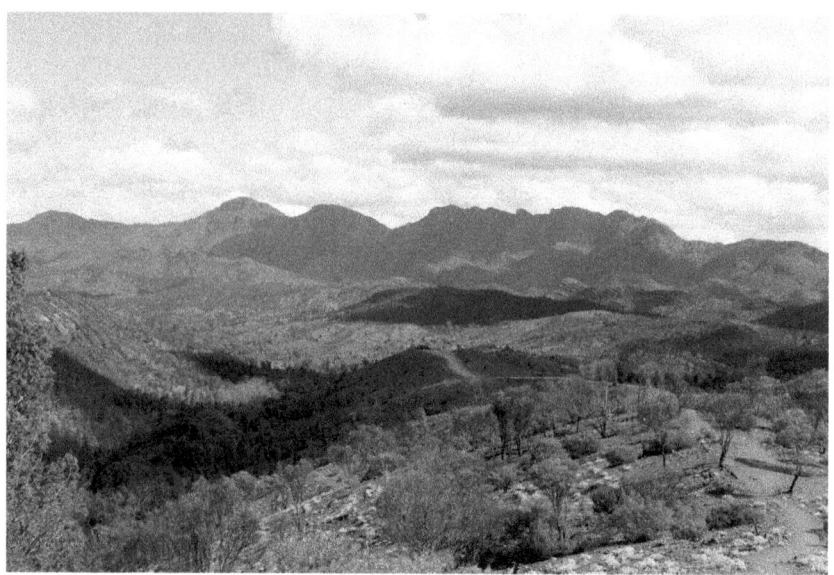

Bunyeroo Gorge

commissioned to survey the boundary between the good rainfall areas and those prone to drought. His survey culminated in what became known as 'Goyder's line': the boundary between reliable cropping land and 'station country' of saltbush and spinifex. Goyder's line closely follows the 10-inch rainfall contour; Carrieton and Belton where the Heaslips congregated were right on the edge of that line.

In the early years, they prospered with cropping and grazing above Goyder's line, but they had the wisdom to consolidate their holdings in the reliable rainfall areas below Carrieton in times of plenty.

The work of Goyder in delineating reliable farming land from semi-desert was not known in the early stages of Heaslip land expansion. In their first two decades of settlement in the Euralia–Belton area (renamed Carrieton in 1894) there were good, if patchy, returns in cropping and grazing. Many farmers in the area abandoned their holdings after successive years of drought. The Heaslips saw this as an opportunity, using funds set aside from the good years to purchase land at a fraction of its previous price.

The Heaslip agricultural dynasty – the story from the diary

Since 1858, the Heaslip families expanded their land holdings from Angle Vale (near Gawler) to Appila and further north to Belton and Carrieton. James and Sophia had moved to Appila, taking advantage of the new land releases and purchasing arrangements passed by the *South Australia Act, 1872*, enabling land to be purchased on credit after a 10 per cent deposit was paid. James Heaslip took up 650 acres in his own name, and Frances took up 98 acres. Together the 748 acres were purchased at a price of £2/6/2 per acre, total £1726. Later there were purchases by James Heaslip in 1882 and William Henry Heaslip in 1908, by which time the Heaslip homeland was consolidated. By 1875 the land had been cleared, fences were being erected and fields ploughed, and the first wheat carted from Willow Park to Laura. On 29 September, 74 bags were carted and in November a further 828 bags; 3384 bushels were sold for £4/1 a bushel. At the time there was a shortage of labour, and contractors (J. Buckley and Son) were engaged to reap for £3/5/0 per week.

Willow Park was approximately halfway between Burra and the copper triangle towns of Moonta, Wallaroo and Kadina. During the 'Monster Mine' period, the population of Burra rose to 5000, making it the seventh largest town in the state. These developments greatly enhanced the prosperity of farming in the region by providing outlets for meat, grain and farm produce for the bakeries, butchers, blacksmiths and light manufacturing facilities in the area. The Heaslips formed a farm implement production facility in Crystal Brook, which also traded in tractors and other farm machinery.

Further north at Belton, William Henry Heaslip was planting wheat and grazing sheep in tandem with his father and family in the Appila (formerly Yarrowie) area. Belton was on marginal land above Goyder's line, but with family cooperation and astute trading Henry and his family prospered. That was not the case for surrounding farms.

At Eurilpa, settlers were selling their farms and James was buying them. During the year he purchased Giddings, McCafferie's for £4/6 per acre, and two other properties at £6 per acre. The tax return forms filled out by James, Sid and Willie in 1885 placed a value on their 'unimproved' lands in Appila of £1000 per acre; the value they placed on 'improved' land was £1500 per acre.

In 1893 James Heaslip died in traumatic circumstances. On 13 November, his wife Sophia and their daughter Fanny started out from Eurelia to take James back to Willow Park 'with Pa very ill'. About 22 miles from Eurelia, at the Euralia Government well, James was in great pain and asked Sophia and Fan to lift him from the cart. They placed him sitting with his back to the stone tank where he rested until he died. Next morning, Sophia and Fan lifted James (a large man) back on the cart and drove the 50 miles on to Willow Park.

Sadly, in that same year, James and Sophia lost their youngest child, eight-year-old Gordon Wyatt. Young Gordon was taken several times to Adelaide with progressive renal disease with anasarca necessitating drainage of fluid from around the lungs. James was buried in the family plot at Appila alongside Gordon, who had been laid to rest just four months earlier.

James had guided the family for 35 years. During that time, he and his siblings established an agricultural estate that was to be a powerful force not only in agriculture but in community service and leadership. That success was marked by hard work in the Wesleyan tradition, families working together with astute financial management.

In 1894, William Henry Heaslip (WHH) married Anna Sweet McDonald (Nan), shortly after the death of his father. Together they settled around Belton where the land was harsh. It was not just the challenge of prospering in a fickle climate but also the hordes of rabbits, plagues of locusts, dingoes, feral cats and dogs, and kangaroos trampling down the crops.

Much of the land in this area was above Goyder's line. In 1890 WHH wrote that the people in the area 'cling to their land with the utmost fortitude, enduring every kind of privation. The hope for better times was their only solace'. WHH and his family, however, prospered almost certainly because of the mutual support provided by his many family members in the Mid and Upper North.

The couple returned to Eurilpa via Adelaide where they purchased furniture and got on with life after dealing with the settlement of James's estate. In 1893 and 1894 there were good rains; at Carrieton they reaped 3750 bushels in 1893 and 3821 bushels in 1894, which they sold in 1896 for an average of £3/10 per bushel. On Christmas Day of 1894 it rained all day for a total of three inches of rain filling all the tanks and dams to overflowing.

In 1895 WHH decided to name his property at Carrieton/Belton Glenroy Estate. In the same year, Nan was expecting their first child who arrived stillborn on 8 August.

The year 1885 was the last of the good rain for seven years. This drought, which finally broke in 1903, had an adverse impact on sheep productivity and wheat crops, but with ever-increasing land purchases Henry was able to improve income from wool and stock sales, which somewhat cushioned the poor wheat yields.

In the spring of 1900, the wheat crops were suffering in drought conditions, but were also under constant threat from rabbits, which could wreak havoc on newly emerging crops. It was all hands-on deck to shoot rabbits to prevent a total wipeout of crops. While shooting was essential for controlling vermin, the development of shooting matches was a much-enjoyed sport. Teams competed regularly in country regions and often in Adelaide. Shooting competitions were also national, and WHH even went to Sydney with many shooters to compete at the Randwick Rifle Range. Proficiency at shooting developed more urgency as soldiers were being recruited for the Boer War. WHH saw off the second contingent from Port Adelaide, which included two Heaslips.

WHH and Nan's first son James Alexander Heaslip arrived at 6 pm on 11 October 1900. Their second son, William Gordon, was born on 2 August 1902.

Seasons in subsequent years slowly improved coming out of the seven-year drought. WHH was able to get good prices for wheat, wool and sheep in the neighbouring towns. Most importantly WHH was able to purchase more land around Willow Park in Appila where the seasons were more favourable, the markets closer and schools nearby.

WHH served on the Ororoo/Carrieton Council between 1899 and 1909 and was chairman between 1904 and 1905.

In the late 1880s WHH and family had extensive holdings around Carrieton/Ororoo and were committed to development of the area.

Glenroy to Appila

In 1908, WHH sold Glenroy to George Anesbury and moved the family to Appila on the land that he had been purchasing over recent years. By 1908 WHH's children were approaching school age: Nan had been taking them through home lessons but the move to Appila allowed them to enrol in formal schooling. The children began primary school already well prepared in reading, writing and arithmetic – a great tribute to their mother who continued to guide them in their reading of literature and participation in affairs of the community like town meetings, parties and Methodist gatherings.

This year marked an important development for agriculture, transport and rural productivity. WHH purchased a motorbike, which he rode in the move from Glenroy to Willow Park; this was the forerunner of farm mechanisation with motorised tractors, ploughing, harvesting and transport. The arrival of the motor car changed society; Heaslips were early adopters of technology, and they purchased a Talbot car in 1914, as well as several tractors and trucks. When caterpillar tractors became available, they purchased one to carve out dams on their newly acquired pastoral lease at Gilles Downs adjacent to Iron Knob where sheep thrived on the saltbush.

Appila was consolidated and served as the centre of Heaslip agricultural holdings through the 20th century.

The struggles

The land above Goyder's line was real hardship country. Many of the first settlers struggled through droughts interspersed with years of rain.

Additionally, the initial surveying and land allocations for sale in and around Belton were woefully inadequate, being of one rood (about a quarter acre or 1000 square metres). The Hundred of Euralia was proclaimed in the mid-1860s before government was aware that land in this area was inadequate for farming. These were the circumstances that allowed the likes of WHH to garner large land holdings and 'ride through' the tough times in wait for opportunities to expand their holdings.

By 1900, the Heaslip families had substantial holdings in both the Hundred of Appila and Hundred of Euralia which provided the opportunity for family to work together for harvesting, stock movements, sharing machinery and most important to watch out for opportunities to acquire more land in the reliable rainfall areas in the Mid North. The Heaslips wisely chose to make good their holdings in the Carrieton/Belton area during the good years and transfer their capital and farming activities to the Appila area.

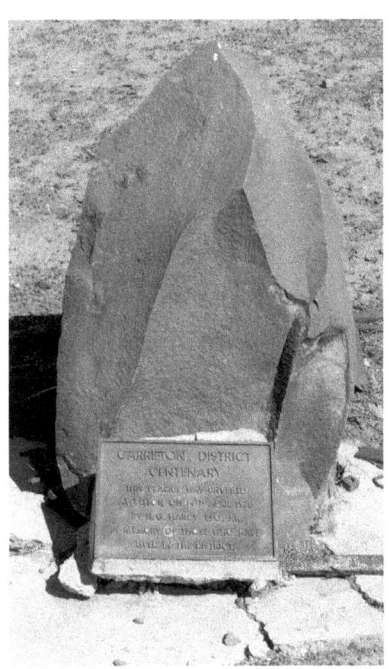

Belton Centenary Plaque

In the century following the establishment of Glenroy in Belton, the productivity of the land decreased in a series of droughts and incremental reductions of average rainfall. All that remains of Belton in the 21st century is a plaque in memory of those who have lived in Belton.

The plaque reads: 'Carrieton District Centenary: this plaque was unveiled at Belton on 14th April 1978 by H.G. Hardy Esq. J.P., in memory of those who have lived in this district. Saltbush thrived in this country and still supports sheep grazing.'

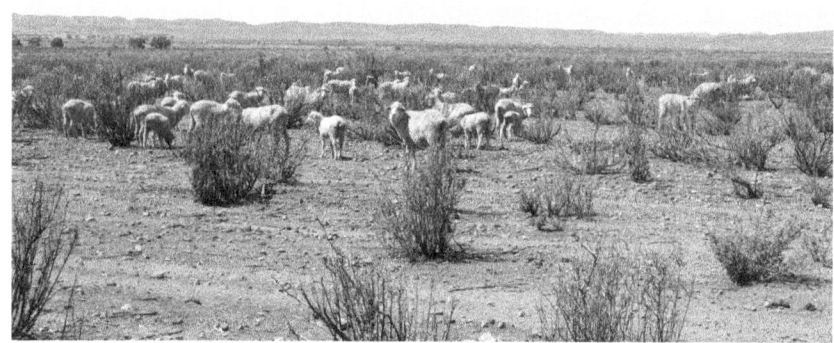

Sheep grazing Belton area

Gordon strives beyond farming

In 1919 the Heaslip land holdings were prodigious, and the family was cited by government as being one of South Australia's first families. For successive generations the clan have been successful in establishing a major agribusiness in South Australia by way of hard work, prudent financial management and utilising a family network to increase output, all while being active participants in community service through local government and their Methodist faith.

As the Heaslip families grew, the children were progressively deployed onto new properties and agricultural pursuits. Gordon had other aspirations. These were formed by his Sunday school and Methodist church experience, outstanding primary and secondary education, and family success in agriculture.

Chapter 2

Pathway to the Missions

Education and aspirations
We do not know exactly when Gordon decided to become a medical missionary. Certainly, as a young teenager he was determined to acquire the education he would require for that vocation – and in achieving that goal he made remarkable efforts. Notably, he was at cross-purposes with his father, who envisaged Gordon completing his primary education and then taking his place in work on the family farm. But Gordon would not comply with these wishes. He was intent on enrolling at Gladstone High School, and valiantly demonstrated his commitment by riding to school each day on his bicycle – over rough roads for many kilometres. Seeing that Gordon was in earnest, Heaslip senior relented, and arranged for his son to board with a relative in Gladstone.

Schooling presented a challenge for the pioneering families. The Heaslips were clearly literate people at the time of settlement. For the first generation in South Australia, home schooling was favoured in providing basic primary school education; Ben senior's children were competent in language, reading and basic mathematics as demonstrated by their ability to maintain the diary, engage in trade, and successfully negotiate land dealings. When WHH developed his first major holdings around Belton and Carrieton the family had to be content with home schooling. The consolidation of the family in Appila provided the opportunity to attend school.

During the latter half of 1876 the first school opened in the town of Yarrowie (now Appila). This school operated as a Protestant Day School; the inaugural teacher James Coane was appointed after receiving a written promise from the residents that they would send at least 33 children to the school, but student numbers dropped from 40 down to an average of 23 by October. The teacher's income was derived from school fees, and he was paid only £9 for the remainder of the year.

In 1877 the Catholic Sisters of Saint Joseph opened a convent school, and later that year the Council of Education completed a school building. This Council of Education was established in 1875 under the Education Act, which introduced compulsory schooling for children residing within two miles of a school. At this time, the government of South Australia had insufficient funds to allocate to education. The task of building schools all over the state was overwhelming, so government gave preference to those districts willing to contribute to the costs of the buildings.

The residents of Appila contributed £100 to the £780 cost of building the school. Concurrently, the SA Government placed grants of land under the control of the Regional Council such that 3000 acres were leased by council to farmers Tinline and Murray from 1877 for a yearly rental of £182. The rent received was used for school construction.

In 1878 the Appila school opened with an Irish immigrant James McClintock teaching 68 children. Payment of school fees continued for children up to 18 years of age until 1892 and for those over 18 years until 1899.

After completing primary school, Gordon sought to proceed with further education at high school, but it seemed that his father might not support his aspirations. Family legend has it that young Gordon rode his pushbike from Appila to Gladstone over 40 kilometres of unmade roads to prove to his father that he really wanted an education. This was until arrangements were established for him to board in Gladstone with his widowed aunt 'Granny' whose husband died in 1881.

Gladstone High School was established in 1907, initially with a 'continuation class' beyond completion of primary school. Alexander A. Heaslip joined the inaugural continuation class in 1907 and was followed by Lizzie M. Heaslip in 1915, then Stella B. Heaslip and Gordon W. Heaslip in 1916. The Gladstone High School was served by a railway and there was a junction at Gladstone that enabled students from a wide area to attend: they came from Crystal Brook in the south-west, Laura and Wirrabara in the north, Caltowie and Jamestown in the north-east and Georgetown and Yacka down south.

This area of the Mid North was prosperous, and the towns had considerable populations (at this time there were more people in South Australia living in the rural and mining towns than in Adelaide and suburbs), so it was not surprising that Gladstone High attracted some of the brightest students in South Australia, including G.R. Fisher in 1925, R.R. St Chamberlain in 1922, and S.B. Forgan in 1926.

Gordon's aspirations at high school
Gordon Heaslip had his sights set way beyond Appila. He was influenced by his faith in Methodism and the knowledge of international markets for farm produce.

For Gordon, further insights into international affairs came from stories based on the Methodist Missionary Society of Australasia who first came to PNG in 1875; by 1927 the books of the mission in Rabaul recorded 313 church buildings, 11 ministers, 227 indigenous pastor-teachers, 9875 scholars in day schools, and 39,020 members and adherents of the church.* Doubtless, lay preachers and visiting church dignitaries promulgated the impact of religion on indigenous peoples. Gordon would have been enthralled by the exploits of Dr Livingstone in Africa and the extensive global missionary movements established in the late 1800s. Gordon resolved to become a missionary in the Methodist faith.

A note in the Heaslip Diaries (p. 76) recounts: 'His father in his wisdom told him that if he was to be a missionary he must also have a profession and that he would have to become a doctor because he was sure he would not remain a missionary.'

---

* Newell Platten, *Hybrid Beauty: An architect, a missionary, and their improbable desires*, Mile End, South Australia, Wakefield Press, 2016.

In 1918 Gordon attended Prince Alfred College for one year, passing the Senior Public Examination which allowed him to progress to university. After matriculation, his father required him to work on the farm to earn the capital to support him through further studies. Capital in this sense was not so much financial but rather 'family capital'. Gordon worked on the farm for four years with no wages before he received parental approval to progress to tertiary education.

Finally, Gordon was then able to pursue his medical missionary training, which involved studies in Theology, a medical undergraduate degree (MBBS) and postgraduate training in tropical medicine.

Ministry training
Gordon Heaslip commenced theological studies in mid-1923 ahead of his enrolment in the Adelaide medical course in 1924. He was the first South Australian to enrol in Medical Missionary studies, which required him to live-in at the Brighton College of Methodist Ministry studies.

As a student of ministry studies, he was required to participate in practical ministry activities that included overseeing the Sunday school at McBride Hall in the Bowden circuit and at Sunday services in the city and country. Gordon came home on holidays and during those times he was involved in lay preaching at the several churches in the Appila circuit.

These ministry responsibilities occurred throughout his medical course, which meant that he was unable to leave South Australia to undertake clinical studies interstate and overseas like many of his fellow medical students.

Gordon was committed to becoming a medical missionary since it fulfilled his boyhood vision of working as a missionary and provided him with an alternative career option. Gordon would also have known that the global Protestant missionary movement had determined that the provision of health and medical services was an effective way of drawing local populations into their evangelising missions. Many medical missions provided medical services to the colonising powers in-country from whom they received financial support. This synergy greatly facilitated colonial expansion because the expatriate populations were prone to tropical diseases and the capacity to receive medical assistance in-country from the medical missions reduced the number of ill expatriates needing to be sent to the 'home-country' for treatment and care. Importantly, the colonising powers brought 'curative' medicine that eradicated or substantially reduced ancient diseases like leprosy, tuberculosis, maternal and infant mortality, smallpox, plague, and many causes of blindness.

These were the reasons that the Methodist Missionary Society sponsored suitable candidates to train in medicine, ministry, and tropical medicine before deploying them to 'The Missions'. Gordon was a diligent student, being awarded the RS Smith prize for his first year of study at Brighton College.

In summary, Gordon pursued a combination of courses that were dedicated to missionary aspirations. This compromised the effectiveness of the medical training to provide the experience and training required for becoming a fully competent doctor. There was no supervised medical internship prior to registration.

The next sections outline how Gordon's medical training was fraught by his religious studies but presented career options for Gordon when his missionary posting failed. He was then able to pursue medical research and fulfil his life ambitions because of the tuition he received in the early years of the medical course.

Gordon's Adelaide medical course, 1924–1929

Gordon commenced his medical course at a time when the Medical School was recovering from a series of misadventures.

The first was the contraction of the course between 1897 and 1901 due to the 'Adelaide Hospital Row' when Adelaide University academics withdrew their services for patient care and teaching which meant that students went interstate or overseas to complete their studies. However pre-clinical teaching continued for all students and provided high-quality teaching and preparation for clinical studies that were often taken outside Adelaide.

In the years after the contraction of clinical teaching there were only 44 graduates between 1904 and the commencement of World War 1 in 1914.

Many students and teachers participated in WWI, which reduced the number of clinicians to provide patient care and teaching after the war.

Following the course disruption from the Adelaide Hospital Row and WWI, medical graduate numbers increased. Between 1926 and 1928, 63 students graduated. When Gordon graduated in 1929 there were nine others in his graduating class.

When Gordon was at medical school, the professors in physiology, anatomy and pathological sciences, and microbiology were people of international renown who enthused their students with discoveries in natural sciences. They presented courses that provided students with a firm basis for future studies in medical science.

Gordon prospered as a student, receiving credits for his studies, and gaining interest in microbiology and natural history as it related to his agricultural background.

University life was more than studying courses towards a degree. Gordon participated in university life as a gregarious country boy with experience in rifle-shooting and outdoor activities in the bush. Riding motorcycles was a favourite means of enjoyment. He received a 'blue' for rifle shooting and participated in motorcycle antics that were commonplace among students. He was renowned for standing on the seat of his motorcycle as a demonstration of prowess but came to grief in an accident with a fuel delivery truck when he slid under the truck and escaped unscathed, a feat reported in the local newspaper.

Pre-clinical sciences

Having spent four years on the Heaslip farms before medical studies,

Gordon was familiar with animal husbandry, plant growth, harvesting and wild animals. The topics of physiology, zoology, anatomy, and pathology were the mainstay of pre-clinical studies and Gordon developed an in-depth understanding of these topics from the teaching and research of the principal lecturers.

These lecturers provided basic teaching in subjects required for clinical medicine and they also engaged their students in research and university life that incentivised future careers in medicine and science. A number of lecturers influenced Gordon Heaslip's career.

Edward Stirling, lecturer in physiology was a surgeon with interests in South Australian fauna. In 1890 he travelled with South Australia's Governor, Lord Kintore, from Port Darwin to Adelaide and collected unique Australian species including the southern marsupial mole [*Notoryctes typhlops*]. He also reconstructed from fossil bones the complete skeleton of *Diprotodon australis,* the four-metre-long marsupial that co-existed with Aboriginal people and became extinct 25,000 years ago. He then partially reconstructed an immense wombat and a bird allied to the New Zealand moa. Five new species of lizard were identified.

Stirling was appointed Director of the South Australian Museum from 1884 to 1912, and he established the infrastructure in SA natural history that supported Gordon Heaslip in medical research in North Queensland.

J.B. [Bertie] Cleland, Professor of Pathology, and microbiology from 1920 to 1940 at the University of Adelaide, established courses in pathology and microbiology alongside his pursuits as a naturalist and collector of new species of plants, animals and fungi.

Cleland is renowned for conducting, demonstrating and writing about large numbers of autopsies that provided students with insights into disease processes that were poorly described in texts of the day. He left his collections to the SA Museum and is memorialised by the foundation of Cleland Park in the Mt Lofty Ranges.

Cleland was primarily a microbiologist and taught the identification of bacteria in the pathology of infectious diseases.

Archibald Watson was the inaugural Professor of Anatomy who served for 34 years. He was a gregarious character who was the only academic to continue providing teaching and clinical services as surgeon when all other clinical academics withheld their service. He taught pathology as well as anatomy and enthusiastically supported students in their studies and socialising.*

The following incident is cited in Gwyn MacFarlane's biography, *Howard Florey: The making of a great scientist*:

> *It happened that a famous anatomist was visiting Adelaide and the Dean of the Medical School asked Professor Watson to arrange an interesting demonstration. Watson expressed his opinion of such visitations with his usual pungency, but finally agreed. The visitor and his entourage arrived in the dissecting-room. Watson blew a whistle, and through the double doors roared six motorcycles, including Howard on his Triumph, to perform intricate manoeuvres between the tables.*

More than most, Watson held the medical course together through the difficult years of WWI and academic withdrawal of services. This enabled preclinical teaching to continue and provide the basis for teaching clinical medicine in later years.

Gordon Heaslip excelled in pre-clinical studies, acquainting him with people and infrastructure in pathology and microbiology in Adelaide that later enabled him to pursue a career in medical research.

The clinical years

Teaching and training in diagnosis and management of diseases was limited by the availability of suitable patients, increasing numbers of students, and few experienced clinicians.

---

* R.G. MacFarline, *Howard Florey: The Making of a Great Scientist*, Oxford, New York, Oxford University Press, 1979, pp. 45–46

The Adelaide Hospital provided teaching facilities and staff for topics specified by the medical school as requirements for graduation. Each student was required to keep an attendance record of autopsies, lectures on specific diseases, instruction on surgical procedures and attendance at specialty clinics like ophthalmology.

This record was signed by the Medical Superintendent and Chairman of the Adelaide Hospital Board for each clinical year and was a pre-requisite for graduation.

Gordon progressed through the clinical years and graduated in 1929.

In later years, Gordon believed that he was inadequately trained in clinical medicine and unable to provide care for patients in the community during his time as a medical missionary. He therefore chose to pursue a career in pathology and microbiology rather than routine patient care.

He expressed the view that he suffered as a student at the hands of professors and lecturers who had been given no training as teachers in clinical medicine. Further, he lamented that his clinical teaching was confined to disease management of patients in hospital.

Throughout his medical course he received no teaching about community general practice, prevention of disease or promotion of health.

Why was Gordon Heaslip dissatisfied with clinical teaching?

The primary reason for dissatisfaction was the quality of the teachers and course content.

This problem with clinical teaching was well known and many students chose to pursue clinical teaching interstate and overseas where the teachers were experienced and introduced students to the breadth of medical conditions.

During the years when the Adelaide Medical School provided pre-clinical training only, students completed their clinical teaching interstate and graduated MBBS. In the years after WWI many students chose to complete their training in this way.

Gordon was confined to South Australia because he was required to maintain his commitments to lay preaching and religious studies. This prevented him from travelling away for more comprehensive clinical experience.

He was not alone in being confined to South Australia for clinical studies. Howard Florey and others were kept in South Australia because of the economic downturn. MacFarlane's biography of Florey states: 'Howard passed his pre-clinical exams with honours; he then proceeded with the clinical teaching of medicine which came to him as a shock.'

The formal teaching was straight from standard textbooks (such as Osler's on medicine and Rose and Carless's on surgery), which students were expected to absorb – even memorise, but not digest. On the other hand, it became obvious in the wards that patients persist in being individuals, and that their ailments can rarely be fitted exactly into neat categories. There was a tendency therefore for teachers to gloss over or ignore misfit facts. The best clinicians who relied more on personal judgement and experience than on textbooks were not considered the best teachers. It was clear that the practice of medicine was still an art rather than a science. Howard would have accepted this situation, though he was more of a scientist than an artist, if it had been honestly presented. What he could not accept was an unquestioning attitude to authority and the concealment of ignorance by long words and pompous phrases.

Overall, Gordon enjoyed his university years. In 1925 he met his future wife, Barbara Kate Shorney, a first-year Arts student. Barbara had a notable academic record. In 1924, her last year at school, she won the Tennyson Medal for English Literature, was top student in English I, and graduated BA in 1928.

A devout Wesleyan, Barbara apparently had much in common with Gordon. Her family had an active interest in the Methodist foreign missions; her sister Winifred was librarian of the Missionary Lending Library in Pirie Street, Adelaide.

On 18 August 1929, Gordon and Barbara married before graduation in the final year of his course and moved into his mother-in-law's house in Unley. Mrs Shorney had died suddenly in Winnipeg while visiting Shorney relatives in North America earlier that year.

Gordon was awarded a blue for prowess in rifle shooting and was renowned for his antics on his motorcycle. He graduated MBBS Adelaide on 11 December 1929 in the presence of his family, who journeyed to Adelaide in the Willys-Knight. Like all graduates, Gordon was able to practice medicine after graduation.

In 1930, the Methodist Missionary Society of Australasia prepared Gordon and Barbara for their missionary posting by arranging for them to travel to Sydney. Here Gordon completed a course in tropical medicine and meetings were arranged with fellow missionaries to prepare them for their ministry duties and the assistance they would receive while they were in post.

Chapter 3

Tropical Training, Papua

Papua New Guinea

Gordon and Barbara Heaslip, now aged 28 and 23, found themselves posted to the village of Salamo on Fergusson Island off the east coast of Papua. The territories of British-administered Papua and Australian-administered New Guinea were combined as an administrative union in 1949 when the country became known as Papua New Guinea (PNG).

In 1930, the population of PNG was 1.077 million; in 1940 it was 1.318 million. According to the World Bank, on independence in 1975 the population had increased to 3,139,945 – a modest increase. Between independence and 2016 the total population increased to 8,085,000 (WHO).

When Gordon and Barbara Heaslip were missionaries, the country was called Papua.

Methodist missionary history

In 1804 the British Methodist Conference established a Standing Committee of Finance and Advice to manage its foreign relations and form district auxiliaries to support the work of the overseas missions. This occurred after Thomas Coke, a close associate of John Wesley, visited Antigua in 1786 and sent missions to almost every colony in the West Indies, and then to Sierra Leone (1811) and Ceylon (1813). The British Methodist Conference formally established the Wesleyan Missionary Society in 1818 and embarked on a global strategy.

Methodist missions were set up in the West Indies, Canada, India,

China, New Zealand, the Pacific Islands and Australia. The first Australian establishment was a mission for convicts in New South Wales in 1818, followed by missions established in Van Diemen's Land (Tasmania) in 1821, Port Philip (1840), South Australia (1840), Western Australia (1840) and Moreton Bay (1850).

The Pacific missions were particularly successful in Fiji, where Wesleyans made up almost half of the population, and in Tonga, where Wesleyan Methodism became the official religion of the Friendly Islands.

In 1852 the British Methodist Conference dispatched Robert Young to Australia to work out a plan for autonomy of the Wesleyan Churches. The British Methodist Conference in Birmingham approved the formation of the Australasian Methodist Connexion in 1854. The Australasian Conference took over the Wesleyan missions in the Pacific, and the first Conference took place in Sydney in 1855, where William Boyce was elected as the first president.

A separate New Zealand Conference was established in 1910 and the missions in Tonga, Fiji and Samoa became autonomous in 1964.

In 1932, the Wesleyan Methodist Church, the United Methodist Church and the Primitive Methodist Church united to form the Methodist Church of Great Britain. The missionary societies of the three churches merged to form the Methodist Missionary Society in 1932, which was dissolved in 2013.

Over two centuries the Methodist/Wesleyan movement was a grass-roots movement that evolved into an organisational structure of great complexity that remained true to its founding principles as a community-controlled organisation.

The Methodist Missionary Society of Australasia (MMSA) in 1930 was based in Sydney where it planned, recruited, trained and supported missionaries in post in the Australasia region. MMSA maintained a motor yacht that regularly visited each mission to provide supplies and, importantly, to support the missionaries and their families in post. MSSA was the link between the missions in the field and the Methodist congregations globally. A regular newsletter, *The Missionary Review*, was produced and widely disseminated. This regular information from the mission posts provided vital contacts between the missionaries and their 'home' congregations and was a crucial element in raising the prodigious funds required to support the missions.

Living and working in the tropics

The global strategy for Methodist mission training included provision for medical missionary training. It comprised an undergraduate medical training in conjunction with ministry studies and a post-graduate course in tropical medicine.

In Australia, MMSA had arrangements with the University of Sydney to provide training in tropical medicine for those undertaking medical missionary training. The School of Public Health and Tropical Medicine at the University of Sydney was established in 1930 expressly to serve Australia and its dependencies in the Pacific. The course was funded by the Commonwealth Department of Health and employed staff from the Commonwealth Department of Health, the Commonwealth Serum Laboratories, and non-government organisations. The initial mission for the school was to train people preparing to work in the tropics. These included government officials, missionaries and military personnel. As well as providing tuition in core subjects of public health – epidemiology, hygiene and statistics – the school also provided a postgraduate program in tropical medicine that was affiliated with the course provided by the London School of Tropical Medicine.

Prior to the establishment of the School of Public Health and Tropical Medicine in Sydney in 1930, the only Australian training in tropical medicine was the Australian Institute of Tropical Medicine (AITM).

Tropical diseases

Prior to colonisation of the tropics the major advances in understanding disease arose from the discoveries of Pasteur, Koch and Lister who identified the microbial causes of diseases that were commonly encountered in Europe.

The exploits of early medical missionaries who went to the tropics, primarily to evangelise, brought back descriptions of tropical diseases that were largely unknown to the Western world, including elephantiasis, malaria and 'River-Blindness' (Onchocerciasis). Known infections such as tuberculosis, cholera, pneumonia and smallpox often manifested in more severe forms in the tropics because of environmental factors. Worse still, many common infectious diseases from the Western world including measles, syphilis and the plague were transported to tropical countries.

In 1878, Dr Patrick Manson published his seminal observations on tropical diseases (Manson P. *On the development of* Filaria sanguinis hominis *and on the mosquito considered as a nurse,* J Linn Soc (Zool.) 1878:14:304–311). His findings led to the discovery that many of the diseases manifested in the tropics and sub-tropics were part of a life cycle of infection that involved a vector.

Malaria is perhaps the most important global infection involving an insect vector. There are several species of malaria parasites that infect humans, the most common two being *P. falciparum* and *P. vivax*. The life cycle of malaria parasites requires that they infect both humans and the *Anopheles* mosquitoes sequentially in order for the parasite to maintain its existence.

The tropical environment fosters vectors of parasitic disease to a greater extent than temperate climates; warm humid weather promotes insect proliferation. When the environment is contaminated by excreta, pathogenic microorganisms are likely to survive in the tropical climate, which presents an opportunity for them to be transmitted both by insect vectors and unhygienic practices to humans.

Vector control programs are the mainstay of programs to control malaria, filariasis and Guinea worm disease (*Dracunculiasis*). While medications have been developed to treat and prevent these vector-borne diseases, resistance can emerge to both the chemicals used for vector control and the drugs used for treatment. There is an ongoing challenge to balance the various approaches to disease control in a manner that recognises that over-reliance on one mode of control will lead to resistance; simple methods like medicated mosquito netting around the bed and wearing long-sleeved shirts can be highly effective.

Parasites are not the only or major cause of tropical diseases. Viruses are prominent causes of disease in the tropics with infections like dengue causing widespread infection. Sometimes infectious agents (often viruses) undergo mutations in their genes that cause a variant virus to become invasive and produce disease. A common example is the influenza virus, which can be observed in most species and occasionally when several species come together (like pigs and poultry) there can be an exchange of genes between the different flu strains to create a new sub-type of virus. This new sub-strain of virus can outwit the pre-programmed immune system in humans (or other susceptible animals), which carries 'memory' of the previous type of virus. The initial response to a new subtype of virus is to produce an immune response against the one in memory. This allows the invading subtype to multiply unchecked by the host immune system.

In 1889, Manson set up a private practice and laboratory in London and passed his membership examination for the Royal College of Physicians. He practised at the Seaman's Hospital at Dreadnought, where he continued to advocate for tropical disease awareness while also criticising the methods of teaching about tropical diseases that medical students received. At an address to the St George Hospital of London he said,

> *the course of instruction in general medicine received in this country is utterly inadequate to qualify for tropical practice. I say so emphatically, basing my assertion on my own experience, my own mistakes and what I have seen and still see daily of the mistakes of others.*

The situation with undergraduate medical education in Australia in 1925 was no different to the courses in Britain that Manson criticised, so it was little wonder that the Methodist Missionary Society in Australasia prepared their medical missionaries by sending them to a course in tropical diseases modelled on the London course initiated by Manson some 30 years earlier.

Having sponsored Gordon Heaslip through his undergraduate degrees, arrangements were made by the Methodist Missionary Society of Australasia for Gordon to complete postgraduate studies in tropical medicine at the University of Sydney.

In Sydney, Gordon and Barbara were hosted by family friends including John Wear Burton, who was general secretary of the MMSA in Sydney.

The course in Sydney in 1930 was as up-to-date as any in the world. When Gordon completed his studies, he was duly appointed as a Fellow of the Society of Tropical Medicine and Hygiene at its meeting on 19 March 1931. Gordon was noted as graduating from Adelaide and posted to Papua.

The Society was important not only for its research and courses of instruction, but it maintained a register of Fellows around the world and provided refresher courses and special meetings that covered the major developments in the field and reports on research.

Adelaide to Salamo, 1930

Gordon and Barbara were in Sydney preparing for their posting to Papua New Guinea in the first half of 1930. Barbara returned to Adelaide in March to attend a meeting to farewell Methodist missionaries who were departing for their missionary postings.

Gordon remained in Sydney completing his course in tropical medicine while living at George Brown College. Barbara stayed with the Burtons when she returned from Adelaide after the missionary farewell meeting.

> # FESTIVAL
>
> on
>
> Tuesday, 4th March, 1930
>
> in the
>
> Exhibition Building
>
> ## MONSTER MEETING
>
> at 7.30 p.m.
>
> "Foreign Missions: Are They Necessary?"
>
> **A meeting to Farewell Departing Missionaries to Salamo**
>
> DR W.G. Heaslip and Mrs Barbara Heaslip

The Heaslip Diary records (p. 100) that 'Gordon and Barbara returned to Adelaide in September, and on the 18th, WHH took them to catch the *Westralia* on their way to Papua New Guinea where Gordon was going as a Medical Missionary.'

The history of PNG depicts a country that was rarely visited by Europeans before 1800 and then only by traders and voyagers of discovery who limited their discovery to coastal regions. In the century of empires (1820–1914), commercial interests discovered the spice islands (Indonesia) but it was the 'first world' missionaries that frequently visited the Asia–Pacific during the 1800s and established many mission stations in the South Pacific and Papua/New Guinea. According to author Ellen Kettle in *That They Might Live*, there appears to have been little contact between the missionaries and colonising nations in this area of the world, unlike the association of missionaries with the colonising nations in Africa, India and China.

Salamo is a large village on Fergusson Island, the largest island in the D'Entrecasteaux group just off the south-east coast of mainland PNG. Methodist Papua had a mission station on Dobu Island, and under

Rev. M.K. Gilmour a review was undertaken to determine optimal sites for extension of mission activities. A 'Development Scheme for Papua' determined that activities of the main station on Dobu should be transferred to the larger Fergusson Island and the site of Salamo was chosen to establish a new Training Institution for the Papua district. The institution comprised a central hospital with a doctor and trained nurses who would not only maintain a hospital for the community but would also train Papuan men and women to staff a series of health clinics in the region.

The district hospital was officially opened by Sir Hubert Murray on the 18 August 1926 with many guests in attendance, including Bishop Henry Newton who represented the Anglican Missions. Many came from Samarai town, the administrative capital of Milne Bay Province until 1968. In earlier days it was a trading port and stopover between Australia and East Asia.

The staff had first moved into the Salamo Hospital in April 1924 when the Rev. Wilison Lagi, a Fijian graduate of the medical school in Suva, arrived. In July of 1924 Dr Henry Judkins of Melbourne arrived with his wife together with Sister Jessie Henry.

This hospital was similar in design and function to most hospitals in Europe and Australia at the time, serving populations the size of those in the province of Milne Bay. It would have been the most modern hospital in Papua at the time. Interestingly a spare room was provided in the doctor's house for the occasional staff member who became ill, most frequently with dysentery or fevers, usually malaria.

Dr Judkins resigned after three years, and was replaced by a New Zealander, Dr Fred Williams . He had specialised in ophthalmology and conducted several cataract operations while in Salamo. Removal of a cataract is a highly specialised procedure requiring great skill and supportive care, but it is one of the most miraculous procedures from the patient's perspective. The fact that Dr Williams was able to successfully complete these operations indicates that the hospital equipment and quality of nursing care were equal to any in the world. News of this 'miraculous' surgery spread far and wide, and the patient demand increased to the point that the nurses were required to devote much of their time to surgical patients at the expense of patrol duties, where they conducted health clinics that provided community care.

Dr Williams departed after 12 months of service. Nine months later, Dr Gordon Heaslip and Barbara arrived. They were presented with an (almost) new hospital and doctor's house, and Gordon was supported with trained nurses while Barbara had house help.

The spectrum of illnesses encountered in this Papuan tropical environment was quite different to those commonly encountered in the more populous tropical countries. Vector-borne diseases of malaria and dengue were an ever-present hazard in Papua, but the people were well-nourished and lived in scattered village communities where hygiene was well maintained. The major health problems encountered in the hospital and clinics were trauma, complications of childbirth, diarrhoea, food poisoning and respiratory infections including tuberculosis, which had been introduced by foreigners.

Illness among staff and families was an ever-present challenge. Dr Wilison Lagi was away at the time of Gordon's arrival because of his wife's illness, returning to work after 12 months, and there were three overseas trained nursing staff who were confined to bed for weeks with dysentery. This gave the Papuan trainees a chance to practice what Gordon, and his predecessors, had taught them.

Gordon wrote,

> *I wish you could have seen Penema. She took over as if she had been matron of a hospital. I can't sufficiently praise the ways in which the students have carried on. The boys have been splendid. They even fed the babies on occasion. Tobi has been acting theatre sister right through, and nothing has been forgotten.*

There was a high birthrate among the Papuans. Gordon remarked that 'an epidemic of newborn babies has overtaken the hospital . . . Penema has now become the perfect assistant'.

In late 1932 there was a severe influenza epidemic that spread through the village, killing many people. In a particularly difficult case, Gordon diagnosed tuberculosis in a newborn who died, which meant that someone with active tuberculosis had nursed the child, most probably the mother. This signalled that tuberculosis was abound in the community. In future decades tuberculosis would become endemic; the Europeans over the years had brought a range of infections to PNG that caused havoc among the indigenous population whose immune systems were ill equipped to deal with foreign diseases.

The hospital had a well-equipped laboratory where Gordon spent much time with the microscope inspecting blood films and looking for bacteria, a skill he learned during his medical course from J.B. Cleland and was later to apply to medical research after he left Papua and missionary life.

Gordon on patrol

Medical missionaries undertook 'routine' clinical duties in the hospital and clinic where there were always patients to be cared for; in Papua these routine duties were dominated by the so-called 'epidemic' of newborn babies. For the most part, Papuan women delivered their babies in a village family setting and only sought help from the mission when complications arose. The number of mothers requiring assistance managed to keep the wards full. Since the babies were mostly born in remote villages, complications of pregnancy and childbirth were often well-progressed because of the time it took first to realise there was a problem, and then for mothers and babies to make their way to a hospital or clinic through jungle paths.

Training of local health workers was crucial in bringing the benefits of 'Western medicine' to the indigenous community. After a period of training in the hospital and clinics these health workers staffed the many clinics in the villages. These clinics performed health checks and provided public health services like vaccination and strategies to avoid mosquito bites. When a person was identified with a specific health problem that required medical attention they would be guided to the hospital and/or clinic. Central to this outreach service provided by the hospital were regular patrols.

Gordon Heaslip provided an account of a patrol he undertook in 1932; it was published in the *Missionary Review* in April of that year. This monthly publication is invaluable for providing information to the congregations in developed countries supporting the missions. It was also an important way for missionaries in the field to communicate with friends, family and congregations back home. The Methodist Missionary Society of Australia was diligent in supporting the members of the faith who had chosen to go to the 'missions.

The article written by Gordon is below:

The Everlasting Hills
A Description of a patrol on Fergusson Island, Papua

Mr Dixon [fellow missionary] and I had been contemplating for a considerable time a trip that would take us through the Gwabigwabi hills, or perhaps they should be dignified by the term mountains. But it is not easy for two people who are moderately busy with different tasks to be able to get away for a fortnight at the same time. However, after several suggested times had proved unsatisfactory or impossible we began preparations to leave Salamo on September 1.

Perhaps I had better say a few words here about preparations for a patrol trip in this country, since it caused me, at any rate, some little worry. The first requisite is natives to carry, and it was herein that I had some trouble. It was a time when natives are busy in their gardens, and at such times love might but money will certainly not get them to go away.

We had only three work boys at the hospital at the time, and one of these had to stay to keep up the essential services. For a fortnight's outing, even travelling as light as we did, one requires a fair amount of impedimenta. To start with, one's sleeping place at the best is an uneven wood floor, made from the shell of the black palm trunk. This, besides being hard, is always dirty, and in the cooler air of the hills permits a lot of ventilation. So at least a waterproof is necessary, plus blankets, and mosquito net.

Clothes have to be changed frequently, as if one is not wet by rain one is by perspiration, so, again, despite meagre attire, a considerable amount of clothing is necessary. Incidentally, my attire for walking is hat, singlet, shorts, socks, and sandshoes, or less, never more. Then a certain amount of literature is required, to pass necessarily idle hours, besides the Dobuan Bible and Hymn Book. And last and most formidable is the question of food. This constitutes the bulk and the weight of the greater portion of the luggage. Everything is in tins that can be got in tins, and with only two travelling there is always a certain amount of waste. Meat, butter, milk and jam are the biggest items. Lanterns, kerosene, buckets and cooking implements make up quite a formidable quantity in themselves. One cannot ask a carrier to accept a load that would be possible in flat country, although, as it is, each carries a load up hill and down dale that would wreck a white man twice the size. I had a student with me of course; but he was more than occupied with the medical outfit and his own luggage. For three days before our departure, I made desperate efforts to get carriers to take the place of two who had promised to come, and had not. Finally, in desperation, I had to increase the load of the two work boys, and take a lad and a man who happened to be at the hospital. The lad was all right, but the man was weak-minded, and owing to some anatomical peculiarity, could only walk at about half the pace of a normal individual.

However, at last we got away, no later than an hour after we intended to. This was quite good, apart from the excuses of my troubles. As it is very difficult to get natives started. Mr Dixon was supplying the cook boy, so we each had five retainers.

Soon after leaving Salamo the river needs to be crossed and

re-crossed. If it is a dry time a couple of boys can, and do, carry one across without much difficulty. If, however, there is much volume of water, the current is too strong for them to do this, particularly as the bed is strewn with boulders of all sizes. I have to have a native to hang on to me when the water gets above my hips, and soon after that one needs to swim, and then walk back the distance one has been carried by the current, to the track. I can assure you that one has no choice but to follow the track in Papua if one wishes to make headway.

At the second crossing we waited a considerable time for my broken-down carrier to arrive. To my relief he finally put in an appearance. It was quite evident, though, that I would have to get another to take his place, or we would be in difficulties. Fortunately, at the next village there had been a death, so all the men-folk were at home. One of these was bribed to carry to a certain village further on, where the process was repeated. The broken-down one was returned to the hospital, where shortly afterwards he got dysentery, went quite mad temporarily, and both sisters went down with the same complaint the night we returned, some twelve days later.

That night we scrambled rather wearily up the precipitous track to the village of Bwelupwa. The elevation is about 1500 feet, but do not imagine it is attained in a nice even gradient from sea level at Salamo. Not by any means. The process is one of going up one, two, three or more hundred feet, and then descending just a little less each time. How far we actually climbed to get there I do not know. Of course, here, as elsewhere in life, there were compensations, for on the way up some glorious panoramic views open out around and below one. Thus from almost the top of one fairly vicious ascent one turns to the right and looks away across Hygeia Bay to Sanaroa. A sea of green, a sea of blue, and then Sanaroa. A little further on one comes out to the top of a rise that is partially cleared, and the sea of green goes sweeping away to the left and upwards to the top of 'Oiatabu [literally, 'sacred hill'], out of sight among the ever-changing clouds of mist. It is over six thousand feet to *the top of this mount, and, like a gleaming knife blade, well up its side, a waterfall cuts the eternal green of the forest.*

But we have to push on, for it is bad enough scrambling up the everlasting hills (everlasting in both senses), in broad daylight. But just before reaching Bwelupwa, a glance to the left through a rift in the trees reveals a perfect picture. We are on a ridge, and almost straight below us is a native village, with its picturesque houses and inevitable coconuts, and an equally inevitable pig lie stretched on the ground between the houses. Seen from this angle, it is indeed a charming picture; the clean swept ground terminating abruptly in the dense forest. We sigh, turn, and resume our upward trend with the words of the poet beating in our ears to the throb of our heartbeats, 'Does the road wind uphill all the way?' The answer is a groan as we go on to prove it does.

At last, not the top, but Bwelupwa. Even the hard floor seems soft to our weary limbs, but the boys seen quite undisturbed by their exertions, and soon we have a steaming mug of tea and a plate of bacon and eggs, the latter carried at no small risk, set before us. Before this, however, we have to bathe in a bucket and put on dry clothes, for there is a big difference in temperature at night between Salamo and Bwelupwa. After tea we sit in the fading light enjoying a well-earned cigarette and, watching the mists creep slowly across the lowlands and obscuring from our gaze the whole of the Dawson Straits. We see that the boys have been sufficiently supplied with food, make arrangements for the breakfast, and then sleep.

Next morning we watch while at breakfast the dissolving of the mists that had gathered the previous night, and then finally before our eyes a sea of green, a ribbon of blue, which is Dawson Straits, and beyond, the rising slopes of Normanby Island. A little to the right we look past the Western end of Normanby across the blue sea to the mighty mountains of the mainland, just visible through the morning haze. Turning our eyes to the left, they travel down the coast of Normanby to the eastern end of the Dawson Straits, where Dobu lies, almost forbidding, with the scarred sides of the extinct volcano that it is, showing forth in the slanting rays of the sun. Going beyond Dobu we follow the coast right down to Bwaruada, and beyond that lies sea and mystery.

But we must be getting on for the day ahead is somewhat worse than the previous one, having only this compensation, a downhill track at the finish. Then there is more trouble. The lad I brought has quite a bad attack of fever, obviously we cannot go on like he is, and equally obvious we cannot wait for him. So we give him into the care of the policeman, with instructions to deliver him to the nearest missionary (native) as soon as he is fit to travel.

We are fortunate here in getting replacements for my carriers, and getting extra ones too, for the track ahead of us is truly bad. Actually our trek lies across a series of converging ridges running from the sea inland and upwards, to form the slopes of 'Ooitabu. And as ridges they are fairly good specimens coming up so precipitously on either side, that the top is quite often only a couple of feet wide. From Bwelupwa we continue upwards along the top of the ridge of the previous evening for about a mile, and then turn to the left slightly, and proceed to cross ridge after ridge more or less at right angles. Most of them are too steep to go straight up or straight down, and occasionally advantage is taken of the meeting of two ridges to avoid going down into the depths. The final result is a track that zig-zags in two planes, and for the traveller considerable weariness of the flesh and irritation of the mind. It really is disheartening to top a long strenuous climb, only to see the track descending into the depths again.

As we continue the ground gets wetter and wetter, and the undergrowth thinner and thinner, until finally we are squelching through mud between giant trees, so closely placed that it almost twilight. There are no people here. We left the last village behind soon after leaving Bwelupwa, and one is given over to muttering missionary and other imprecations on the everlasting hills, and paying a silent tribute to the natives who first tracked their way through the unbroken forest. And now we descend to another creek, between two ridges, and look in vain for a track on the other side. At last we decide there is none, and turn up the creek, stepping from stone to stone in a futile endeavour to keep out of the water. It is quite absurd because our feet are already soaking wet and the stones are treacherously slippery, and each step increases our irritation.

Then quite suddenly we turn out of the main stream up a channel worn by the water through the earth and underlying rock. There is no choice about where one walks here, as the bottom of the channel is only about one to two feet wide, and the sides are about six to eight feet high, and practically vertical. Besides we are going up again at a grade of one in one so we have to save our breath and energy. At last we come out on top of yet another ridge, and now the undergrowth is getting thick again. After a few more ups and downs we start down a long descent, sometimes on our feet and sometimes using our unfortunate shorts for toboggans. It terminates in a creek that is quite a creek, about fifteen yards wide and studded with huge boulders. Here we rest for a while, while the boys refresh themselves with a dip in the cool clear water. With thanksgiving we notice a garden on an adjoining hillside, and know we are once more near habitation. We are; but the ascent from that creek seems to be the longest and steepest for the day. But all things end and we soon break out of the forest into a village. It is dirty and tumbledown, but we do not care, for we know we have temporarily finished with the everlasting hills.

After a rest and a cup of tea we leave the village and start down along a ridge that runs almost down to the bit of level ground running back from the shore. Just here a carrier in the lead takes a wrong turning, and as in moral stories disaster overtakes him. There is a crash as his load hits the ground, and proceeds to follow him as he slides down on the broad of his back. We are greatly cheered by this misfortune in another, being still human, though missionaries.

I must digress here to say that only once before or since have I seen a native fall while carrying, and I have been over many and bad tracks in that time. One more ascent and a gradual descent, and we reach the sea. A comparatively short walk along a shingly and exceedingly meagre beach, at time it ceases to exist at all, and we come to Basima, and the village of Billy, the uncrowned but acknowledged king of that region.

Billy meets us with an air and a handshake, and introduces me (Mr Dixon had already had the honour) to his daughter, Marama. Billy himself is a small man, even for a Papuan, very straight and slim, with a hideously pock-marked face. He is one of the victims and survivors of an epidemic of smallpox that swept the group about 40 years ago.

The history (of Billy) is a story in itself, and if one accepts his statements, a rather lurid one. However, it can be considerably discounted, as even among Papuans Billy is outstanding as a liar. Even so, he has undoubtedly seen, and been the author of, some dark deeds. He tells with great relish the story of how he once convicted a woman of witchcraft, and thereupon tied her to a tree in the village, and left her there till she died. On the other hand, he is rather sensitive about the fact that he had once been the policeman in that district, and had his office taken away by the Government because he was using it to increase his harem. At present he has but three wives. If questioned about this subject of his lost high estate, he breaks forth (if you are a stranger) into a torrent of broken and mutilated English, probably the only part of which you will understand is the considerable stock of English swear words which he has acquired. Soon after our arrival the policeman came along and was instructed to get all the people together for medical treatment and service next morning. He explained that he would do this, but he had to leave early next morning to build a house in another village. We thought this suspicious at the time, but our thoughts were diverted by Billy telling us that we would do much better to leave the policeman alone and consult him about any matter we wanted attended to.

Next morning, we realised why the policeman had had such important business elsewhere. About ten people, all of Billy's village, turned up. We found out, on enquiry, that the people had been told that I was a Government officer and a bad character, and they would be well advised to stay away. They did.

At our last visit we had about 200 men to service. This is one of the disappointments that go to make up a large part of a missionary's life.

That afternoon we contented ourselves with a short distance, as the country was new to us, and it is almost impossible to get information as to distances from natives. The policeman at Basima who knows some English, assured us it was only an hour's walk to the next village, and to prove it, told us that if we left at one o'clock, we would arrive at 12.30 the same day. The track was good and over level ground, and that night we reached and stayed at Gamweta.

Just before reaching the village there is a tiny creek, which makes a break in the forest just sufficient to give a view of a beautiful waterfall about a mile away. From here only the two upper portions of the fall are visible. Next morning I left Mr Dixon to his language researches and walked up to the falls. They are very pretty, but owing to the density of the forest and the precipitous nature of the ground, one can only get a view of the two lower falls. At the foot a deep pool has been worn in the solid rock by the falling water, and this pool is overhung by an immense boulder about ten feet high. It makes an ideal spot for a bathe, as several small boys demonstrated to me by pushing one another off the rock. The village of Gamweta is a pretty spot, with 'Oiatabu rearing its head in the background, and out to sea the Amphletts nestling in their bed of blue. I took advantage of the short walk to this place, and did a little washing in the adjacent creek. I would have enjoyed the performance more had the creek looked a *little less ideal as a home for crocodiles. One has ever to keep in mind the possibility of the presence of these nasty creatures in Papua.*

Next day we walked along the coast to Wadelei. Here we had a reminder of the past, as in one place the ridges of 'Oiatabu run right down to the sea. A little further we came upon another waterfall quite close to the track. It is not as big as the one at Gamweta which can be seen quite a way out to sea on the way to Kiriwiua, but it is a very pretty spot, and one to which people in civilised lands would travel quite a long way for the doubtful pleasure of having a picnic in the proximity.

At Wadelai we were met by Mosese, the Rotumaqn missionary at Salakahadi. This fine man has a huge and hard district to serve around Salakahadi, but has still found the time to visit the otherwise untouched portion of the island. As a result of his labours, we held services at three centres – Wadalei, Bosalewa, and Masemase – taking up the annual native offering to mission work.

The Government resthouse at Wadelai was new and rather artistic in construction. As we were admiring it the discreet and youthful policeman from Basima arrived for reasons best known to himself. We greeted him, and Mr. Dixon remarked, 'Very nice house, this one,' and the answer came pat, 'Very nice too'. We were too polite to laugh then, but did later, when Mr. Dixon diagnosed the case as 'an ex-cook-boy from a place where there had been white women.'

Do you know Simulium? If you have met the little beasts you will not have forgotten them. They are to be found in nearly all the coastal regions of this group of islands and are a particularly vicious type of sandfly. They lost no time after our arrival, and as soon as I discovered what it was that was biting me, I fled incontinently and unashamedly to the inside of the rest-house. It is one of God's mercies that they do not bite in the shade or at nighttime, as a mosquito net is quite useless against them. Mr. Dixon is one of those rare and fortunate people whom they do not affect.

Next day we travelled on to Bosalewa, and held a service there, and I must admit that there were nearly as many dogs there as people. It was decidedly incongruous in the middle of the service to hear an annoyed inhabitant loudly voice his opinion of the dogs. That night we were troubled by mosquitoes, and despite the heat, were glad to retire under our nets. Boselewa is practically at sea level, and is shut in on three sides by hills, and on the fourth by a three to four mile strip of mangrove swamp. We were glad to leave it the next morning, although it was Sunday. At noon we came to a considerable river bed, although the amount of water was small. As the water that flows out here comes from as far away as the watershed between Salakahadi and Galubwa, one can understand that in wet weather there is need for a large channel. Just beyond the river we came to Masemase and held our third thanksgiving service.

At this time I had found no work for the medical unit, as the rumours we met at Basima had preceded us with very evident results.

That afternoon we pushed on to Gwabigwabi hills, a strange site in this land of luxuriant and rank growth. Except for a stunted tussocky kind of coarse grass, they are quite bare. Here also we had trouble with the language, for the policeman's knowledge of English was exceedingly sketchy and his knowledge of Dobu was even less. However, we finally made him understand that we required some carriers and his guidance the next morning. Apart from the fact that it would be hard, hot work climbing the ridges ahead of us, we were in blissful ignorance of what lay ahead. We were about to enter country that no missionary had previously visited, and next morning made an early start, as we were quite ignorant of where we would find shelter for the night.

The first half-mile was all right and brought us to the foot of the hills. The next half-mile was a matter of one foot forward and half a foot up on the average. At times it was one foot forward and two feet up. This little effort brought us out onto a tiny plateau from which we could see the whole of Hughes' Bay, all the Amphletts (a group of scattered islands), and only the haze prevented us from seeing Kiriwina away to the north. After a rest we exemplified 'Excelsior' minus the snow and ice. Just beyond this point we came out on the bare hills, and the track was so hard, steep, and slippery, that Mr. Dixon found it impossible to progress in his boots, and had to take them off. The ground was scorching hot, and the result for Mr. Dixon was a huge blister on each foot. I sympathised with him, but not to the extent of offering him my sandshoes.

We toiled on and up and on and up for what seemed like an interminable distance, and then suddenly forgot all about the heat, the track, and even sore feet, for we were standing on the edge of an almost sheer precipice, dropping down a thousand feet or more to the valley below. To our right it sloped down to the sea, while to our left it rose up and up almost abruptly, curving to the right in the distance and terminating in the slopes of the opposite side. The head of the valley was blocked, as it were, by the same cliff face running right up to the top of a three-thousand-foot peak, which in the distance seemed to come to a point.

Just on the left of the peak on the opposite side of the timber and undergrowth began again, and even from where we were could hear the murmur of the waterfall that dropped into the valley below. Truly it was an awe-inspiring sight, and mercifully we were ignorant that our track ran right over the top of that distant peak. The opposite side of the valley consisted of a grass-grown slope that that rose gradually (for Papua) to the hills beyond. From where we were standing we looked down on to a village on the other side of the valley, and although we could hear the voices of the people there, they looked like Lilliputians in a Lilliputian village. From there we mounted a series of ridges running at right angles to the face of the cliff and to the track. The top of the first of these we named Suicide Point, for we learned that in the olden days it was the custom of the people in disgrace to throw themselves from this spot to certain death

> *below. I suppose this spot was chosen, as the drop is absolutely vertical for some hundreds of feet.*
>
> *After toiling upwards for another mile, we saw the leading carriers emerge on top of the peak, and then there dawned on us the realisation that we were doomed to the pleasure of the whole valley, from its head with a 1500 foot drop immediately in front of us. We finally reached the top and found it to be six yards wide and covered with boulders. It was worth the climb, though it is not one to be repeated frequently.*

From this point the patrol party descended to Salamo, utterly exhausted but enlivened by the glorious perspectives in scenery and adaptation by the indigenous people to this bitter-sweet country.

This 'Missionary Patrol' illustrates the challenges facing foreign settlers in penetrating the tortuous and unforgiving landscape of Papua. It was not until after WWII and the arrival of more modern aircraft that the highest reaches of the highlands were breached.

Health status in Papua, 1930

The population of PNG was comparatively small at 1.077 million and most of this population was living in small villages. The major Government hospitals were in Port Moresby and Samarai, an island in the Milne Bay province adjacent to Salamo. Samarai was a trading port on the shipping lane between Australia and Southeast Asia.

The data on population health in 1930 can be estimated from 1950 data [WHO] when life expectancy at birth was 38.31 years. Reduced life expectancy was due to maternal mortality, failure of infants to thrive after childbirth, and causes of mortality and morbidity that occurred among indigenes in isolated villages. These included infestations with hookworm, yaws that caused pustular sores in young people, pig-bel that occurred after ingestion of days-old pig meat with toxins that caused gut perforation, trauma, and kuru. Additional disease occurred from imported infections including smallpox, Tuberculosis, measles, and sexually transmitted infections.

Malaria was present in Papua before European settlement and over time the population developed a measure of resistance. Europeans are immunologically naïve to malaria and likely to come down with a severe infection in contrast to the natives.

In 1930, little could be provided to treat the clinical symptoms of the diseases intrinsic to Papua, but hygiene [e.g. pit toilets], avoidance of mosquitoes and safe food handling practices were able to diminish the severity of some of these diseases.

Government support for health in 1930 was limited by the economic circumstances of the Depression and limited to provision of a Chief Medical Officer and three or four medical officers and nurses.

General health, pregnancy, trauma and preventive health
The foregoing examples of health status and disease were probably not encountered by Gordon Heaslip during his posting in Salamo.

During his posting at Salamo, Gordon indicates that most medical care and health prevention revolved around pregnancy, childbirth and infant failure-to-thrive.

The sophisticated infrastructure of the Methodist Hospital was equipped to deal with 'European' health conditions, yet was rarely used for this purpose.

Apart from a mention of tuberculosis in the hospital there is little evidence that the Salamo Hospital managed health conditions among Papuans beyond pregnancy and infant care. There is no mention of the diseases associated with morbidity and mortality that contributed to low life expectancy among the Papuans. There were no attempts at preventive medicine beyond visitations on patrol.

For Gordon, his clinical practice was limited and not intellectually challenging despite his extensive training in tropical medicine. However, he used the laboratory facilities and maintained correspondence with fellow medical missionaries who were treating major disease outbreaks and conducting research on vector-borne diseases.

Financial support for the missions was diminishing. In 1933 when the hospital was faced with an epidemic of fever, sores and dysentery among neonates, there were insufficient funds to purchase milk supplements. An attempt to substitute coconut milk for 'lactogen' failed to blunt the epidemic and this situation contributed to a feeling of helplessness among staff. Staff were again tested when influenza afflicted patients and staff alike, but commitment to achieving the best outcome possible enabled the health workers to keep going. What else could they do?

After five years in Salamo, Gordon was disaffected with being a medical missionary.

The hospital had not fulfilled its role as providing the Western medical care it was built for, the village people were unwilling to come to hospital in time for the hospital to provide safer childbirth and prevent the infant morbidity, and Gordon was unable to provide preventive health for the population he was serving. He was keen to pursue medical research, which would give him an opportunity to engage in medical practice and contribute to improving health by way of research on people living in the tropics.

Vale Salamo
During their posting to Salamo, Barbara returned to Adelaide in February 1933 for the birth of their first son Jeffrey, which Gordon attended. The young family travelled back to PNG and stayed for 18 months until October 1934, when Gordon received news of his father's imminent death. They journeyed to Australia, and William Henry died on 1 November.

The couple stayed in Australia until the birth of their first daughter Jocelyn in January 1935 and returned to Salamo for six months before finally leaving PNG for good.

For Gordon and Barbara, Fergusson Island was a hardship posting in many aspects, not just for the burden of tropical life but also the challenges of establishing 'Western medicine' among a population whose knowledge of health and hygiene was severely lacking by Western standards. A proposition to deliver 'best care' in the Western medical tradition in a tropical setting among nomadic indigenous tribes was destined to be fraught.

There was no sadness in leaving as they returned to Adelaide and a new life.

Chapter 4

Research Career, South Australia

Vale Papua and missionary life

In October 1935 Gordon resigned from his missionary post in Salamo. A report from 1936 by the Department of (Methodist) Overseas Missions recounts:

> *The period of economic pressure through which we have been passing has exacted a hard toll from many overburdened men and women in the field.*
>
> *Papua has suffered grievously by the absence of ten members of the white staff on sick leave or furlough. The district lost the services of Dr. Heaslip, who had to retire from the mission through ill-health. His management of the Salamo Hospital and the medical patrol exhibited conspicuous ability. The severe economies of recent years have entailed much sacrifice and patient endurance.* *

Gordon was a proud and competent medical practitioner who kept abreast of world advances in health care through his continuing fellowship of the Society of Tropical Medicine and Hygiene. He acknowledged that conditions in Papua were unable to match his aspirations to advance the health of the indigenous people.

Diseases regarded by Europeans as health problems were considered by Papuans to be part of life and the result of external forces, be they spirits, witches or deities. Children born with disabilities rarely survived into adulthood. There were some infectious diseases observed by

---

* Jocelyn Preece, *Adelaide Woman: A 20th century story: the life and times of Barbara Shorney Heaslip*, Northcote, Victoria, Ghost Words, 2007.

the missionaries that were the result of cultural and food preparation customs that were seen as influenced by the spirit world and accepted as part of life. The notion of (transmissible) infectious diseases was unknown to the indigenous peoples, as were hygiene and safe food preparation.

The Methodist Missionary Society built Salamo Hospital as a demonstration hospital with the most modern healthcare facilities and a commitment to train the indigenous people in up-to-date (Western) medicine and health care. This vision evaporated as financial support dwindled and committed staff struggled to maintain high standards of care despite huge personal investment. Gordon wrote, 'there is justification for the feeling that one is not in any way to blame for these mishaps [inability to feed the babies and outbreaks of dysentery among staff], and that if one had the equipment and facilities, they could be limited'.

Returning to South Australia

The family chose to settle in a stately home in Linden Park, Adelaide. From this prestigious address Gordon and Barbara set about renewing acquaintances in Adelaide and the countryside where Gordon was born. They journeyed to the Heaslip properties in the Mid North at Appila, in the Flinders Ranges at Belton, and the pastoral property of Gilles Downs outside Iron Knob via Whyalla.

After years of tropical secondment as missionaries during the Depression, disenchantment with religion and the challenges of raising two young children on Fergusson Island in Papua, they were ready to explore the world. Within a few months the young Heaslip family was invigorated and eager to gain insights into world affairs. Barbara and Gordon were determined to visit Canada, where Barbara's mother died in 1929. They also planned to visit Britain at the time of the coronation of King George VI to satisfy Gordon's curiosity about the countries Gordon learned about during his farming days.

Once the family had settled in Adelaide and Gordon had considered future career options in South Australia, Barbara and Gordon planned their overseas itinerary. Jeffrey and Jocelyn were left in the care of young nanny Lorna while Gordon and Barbara set off on their world tour.

The liberated Heaslips first journeyed to the United States to visit Barbara's relatives in Chicago. After North America, they travelled to Britain. In London they enjoyed the social life that surrounded the coronation of King George VI. They returned in late 1937 to join their children at their Adelaide home. Jocelyn recalls that her mother returned with tales of grandeur and joy; she admired the elegant evening wear and was enchanted by stories of concerts and dinners that her mother recounted.

Gordon considers the next phase of his career

While in Papua, Gordon learned that the profile of tropical diseases he encountered in Papua differed from those described by colleagues in Africa, India and Asia. During his missionary posting he maintained contact with Fellows of the Society of Tropical Medicine and Hygiene, and scientific journals that outlined the significant advances in the pathogenesis of infectious diseases, particularly those associated with fevers and the role of insect vectors in transmitting diseases. These fevers occurred in locations where humans explored and exploited native bushlands in a manner that provoked insects who were living symbiotically with wild animals to bite and infect humans with previously unknown microbes from wild animals. Gordon decided to build upon his medical experience in Papua and investigate new types of infectious diseases from a base in Adelaide – if possible.

Fortuitously, while Gordon and Barbara were in Papua, and immersing themselves in international developments during their world tour in 1936 and 1937, opportunities arose for considering medical research based in Adelaide.

The economic circumstances and community welfare in Australia changed considerably in the time that Gordon spent working in Papua. The health system had undergone considerable change following the

Great War and the infectious diseases that flourished in its wake. The Spanish Influenza pandemic accompanied returning troops in 1918 at a time when Australia lacked a coordinated national health system. It was not just influenza that burdened the health of the nation. Tuberculosis, unemployment and economic depression coupled with the mortality and injury of young people from war all combined to blunt national productivity and cause a lowering of birth rates for the decade after the war.

Following WWI, the state and Commonwealth departments of health failed to agree on strategies for health prevention of outbreaks of disease, so major national health issues like maternal and child health and vaccine preventable infections went unattended.

In 1925–26 a Royal Commission on Health was conducted to report on coordination of public health between the Commonwealth and states. This resulted in formation of a Federal Health Council that comprised the Commonwealth Director-General of Health and Chief Health Officers from each state, but this council failed to achieve its goals.

In 1937, the Commonwealth Government addressed the problems of national health arising from disparate state health systems by forming the National Health and Medical Research Council (NHMRC), which had two principal aims: to achieve national coordination of public health matters between the states and Commonwealth governments, and to establish a national system for medical research.

The Commonwealth Government established a funding mechanism in perpetuity (Medical Research Endowment Fund) for NHMRC to sponsor research through grants for specific projects and areas of research, as well as training awards and fellowships that enabled medical scientists to pursue a career in medical research.

The establishment of the NHMRC in 1937 coincided with Gordon Heaslip's return to Australia. In Adelaide, the Institute of Medical and Veterinary Sciences had embarked on medical research projects funded by NHMRC, providing Gordon the opportunity to enter the medical research field. He brought with him previous experience in Papua, where he had established a small laboratory in which he performed microscopic and chemical tests on patient samples. At the Institute of Medical and Veterinary Sciences, Gordon took the opportunity to investigate new causes of infection among a group of scientists and institutions in Adelaide that had already established expertise and infrastructure to investigate new infections.

Between 1920 and 1940 Adelaide attracted a number of scientific luminaries in the fields of natural history, microbiology and entomology. The first significant appointment was when J.B. Cleland became the inaugural Marks Professor of Pathology (which then included bacteriology) at the University of Adelaide in 1920. T. Harvey Johnston, as Professor of Zoology, joined Cleland in 1922.

Together they published widely on parasitic diseases in humans, animals and plants. In Adelaide they expanded the laboratory infrastructure for research into vector-transmitted diseases in humans and animals; this included the South Australian Government Laboratory of Pathology and Bacteriology at the Adelaide Hospital, Veterinary Laboratories of the SA Department of Agriculture and the South Australian Museum.

By 1930, the South Australian Museum had a prodigious collection of material contributed by Cleland and Johnston. When Herbert Womersley, an English entomologist, joined the SA Museum, he completed a circle of expertise in Adelaide that pursued research in vector-borne diseases. This group discovered a range of new spiders and insects, and explicated their role in disease of humans and animals. Their publications gained international recognition and collectively established Adelaide as a centre of excellence in natural history. Under the patronage of this group, many aspiring medical scientists underwent training in research and progressed to national scientific and medical leadership.

As well as sponsoring research, this group greatly enhanced the standing of South Australia as a place of international renown in the study of natural sciences and medical research. The explicit role of this group, referred to as the Adelaide Centre of Excellence in Natural History 1920–1940 (ACENH), deserves further recognition.

At the end of 1937, the state government merged the SA Government Laboratories of Bacteriology and Pathology at Adelaide Hospital (SAGLBPAH) and the Veterinary Laboratories of the SA Department of Agriculture into a single institution: the Institute of Medical and Veterinary Sciences. The IMVS was situated in a new building on the grounds of the Adelaide Hospital and brought together the study of human and animal diseases in a single institution in accordance with the *Institute of Medical and Veterinary Science Act 1937*. Originally a government institute, the IMVS became an independent organisation responsible to parliament.

IMVS remained affiliated with the University of Adelaide and appointments to the IMVS received academic recognition by the university. Many IMVS senior staff undertook teaching and research roles as university academics.

The IMVS continued to provide a diagnostic laboratory facility for humans and animals. Initially it performed pathology testing for the Adelaide Hospital and the Department of Agriculture, and progressively expanded its activities as the health and agricultural industries developed. From its inception however, the central focus of the IMVS was research.

Gordon Heaslip began his career in medical research by studying bacteriology at SAGLBPAH. The discipline of bacteriology was regarded as a section of pathology that also included biochemistry, haematology, histopathology, and morbid anatomy. Gordon was taught by Nancy Atkinson in the diagnostic bacteriology laboratory, performing microscopy and culture studies on patient specimens to investigate the cause of infection.

After completing his bacteriology laboratory training, Gordon was awarded a scholarship by NHMRC as research assistant to gain experience in clinical research at the IMVS.

The first annual report of the IMVS Council for 1938–39 acknowledged that doctors W.G. Heaslip and C. Swan were working under the Medical Research Council of the NHMRC and were afforded facilities for their research. In subsequent years they were joined by Neville Stanley and J.M. (Barb) Dwyer as NHMRC research assistants. Gordon's initial research was investigating poliomyelitis, more commonly known as polio.

The first outbreak of polio in South Australia occurred in the early 1920s. In 1922 it was proclaimed an infectious disease alongside other notifiable diseases including diphtheria, measles, scarlet fever and whooping cough. In the same year, the *Metropolitan Infectious Diseases Act* was passed. A new hospital, the Metropolitan Infectious Diseases Hospital, was opened on 7 October 1932 in Northfield. The hospital initially catered for 150 patients in various wards but with the capability of supporting more beds when circumstances demanded. A crisis emerged in 1937 when diphtheria ravaged the community, leaving very few beds for polio patients.

Gordon Heaslip's research on polio explored the possibility that low levels of vitamin C and susceptibility to diphtheria were factors that predisposed patients to contracting poliomyelitis. Gordon implemented a research protocol study which examined 235 patients with polio and a control (comparison) group of patients. His results confirmed his hypothesis that people who were susceptible to infection by diphtheria were likely to suffer a more severe attack of poliomyelitis than control people who were immune to diphtheria (by way of vaccination or previous infection). A similar correlation was found in a study of patients with low levels of vitamin C; patients with low ascorbic acid levels before contracting poliovirus suffered more severely.

In 1938 Gordon published two papers outlining his studies and findings: 'A Case of Relapse in Experimental Poliomyelitis' in *Australian Journal of Experimental Biology and Medical Science*, xvi. 285, and 'Susceptibility to Diphtheria and Vitamin C Nutrition as Possible Factors in the Epidemiology of Poliomyelitis', *Australian Journal of Experimental Biology and Medical Science* xvi. 287. In these reports, he acknowledged that he was working with a personal grant from the National Health and Medical Research Council.

Gordon's research was significant. In the 1930s, polio was a scourge on the Australian population, with hospitals overwhelmed with an enormous number of severely ill adults and children. The people who became ill with polio were only a small proportion of those infected with the virus.

The factors that caused the polio virus to cause disease in otherwise healthy people were largely unknown, hence the global research to look for underlying factors that predisposed patients to serious disease. The factors largely remain conjectural beyond general susceptibility to disease and comorbidities, but Gordon's findings (and others') reinforced the resolve of public health authorities to focus on factors that would prevent the transmission of cross-infection with the polio virus. Gordon's papers were cited by several authors, including MacFarlane Burnet, who were central to leading Australia's response to the polio epidemic.

In the course of conducting this research, Gordon had spent much time working in the bacteriology laboratory and had conducted clinical research. He was now ready to embark on larger research projects that called for expertise at the laboratory and clinical level, as well as the ability to analyse results and publish findings of significance.

Gordon was now qualified to commence clinical research on NHMRC topics of national priority. He was recognised nationally for his success in using laboratory studies to investigate infectious diseases among a group of research scientists within the ACENH who had specialised in vector-borne fevers. This group would become crucial in supporting his future research work in Queensland that required provision of experimental research animals from the IMVS and the expertise of entomologists in the South Australian Museum.

Chapter 5

Queensland and World War II

In 1937, Gordon was interviewed for, and won, a position as chief investigator on a NHMRC grant in Brisbane to investigate the cause of a glandular fever-like illness in North Queensland thought to be a vector-borne disease. Gordon and his family relocated to Cairns for two years, from 1938 to 1940.

Why was Gordon recruited from Adelaide to undertake research in North Queensland when extensive laboratory expertise was present in Brisbane? The most probable reason is Gordon's involvement with the Adelaide Centre of Excellence in Natural History, which had extensive experience and infrastructure to investigate tick-borne fevers and identify new insect vectors.

Coastal fever – the research challenge

In 1934, Sir Raphael Cilento, Director General of Health and Medical Services for Queensland, believed that there were yet unidentified causes of fevers in North Queensland. The fevers resembled glandular fever and scrub typhus, but investigations had failed to identify a specific microbial cause and how such a microorganism might be transmitted to humans. Cilento was aware that scrub typhus, known as tsutsugamushi fever, was reported in Japan after bites from the red spider mite. These Japanese cases occurred mostly along river valleys during floods. The red spider mite, also known as itch mite, was prevalent in North Queensland and PNG, suggesting that coastal fever might be a vector-borne disease.

Most typhus is more benign and generally referred to as 'scrub' typhus because it is transmitted from wild and some domesticated animals to humans by a variety of insects. Scrub typhus is an illness with fever and rash caused by tiny bacteria from the genus *Rickettsia*, which refers to a group of tiny bacteria (0.1μm) that are obligate intracellular parasites – they must live inside host cells. This bacterial genus has been found to be the cause of fevers in various parts of the world.

Rickettsial infections are vector-borne and cause a variety of human diseases ranging from benign to highly pathogenic. Certain species of Rickettsiae were highly pathogenic like *Rickettsia prowazekii*, which caused epidemic typhus and was transmitted between humans by body louse. Since Ricketts first discovered these tiny bacteria as the cause of Rocky Mountain spotted fever, numerous species have been found in different parts of the world associated with species of Rickettsiae that are unique to a particular locale.

In 1935, Cilento pressed Ed Derrick, Director of the Queensland Laboratory of Pathology and Microbiology, to seek funds from the National Health Medical Research Council (NHMRC) to investigate the cause of the fevers in North Queensland. Derrick had success in the past investigating fevers in Queensland. He had discovered a previously unidentified species of leptospirosis (bacterium), *Leptospira pomona*, which infected rats in cane fields, which then excreted infection to canecutters, causing a sometimes-fatal condition recognised internationally as Weil's disease. Subsequently, he investigated the causes of fever among abattoir workers in the Brisbane region, identifying intracellular bacteria in samples from febrile abattoir workers. Derrick designated this disease Q fever, because the microorganisms they observed were unlike any described species. He then forwarded these microorganisms to Sir Frank MacFarlane Burnet and Mavis Freeman at the Walter and Eliza Hall Institute, who characterised the intracellular microorganisms as a new species and named it *Coxiella burnetii*.

Coastal fever was more widespread and clinically different from Q fever, which was transmitted to humans by ecto-parasitic ticks of cattle and pigs and progressed to an atypical pneumonia, and Weil's disease caused by leptospires from infected rodents urinating in cane fields.

Was there a novel microorganism and vector associated with Coastal fever? The application to NHMRC therefore proposed a study with the following objectives (*Medical Journal of Australia*, 2, 22, 555, November 1940):

1. To isolate the strain of *Rickettsia* responsible for the cases of typhus.
2. To identify the vector or vectors of the *Rickettsia*.
3. To discover which of the local fauna act as the reservoir for typhus.
4. To determine whether Q fever exists along the coast of North Queensland.
5. To resolve the nature, cause and epidemiology of any previously unrecognised fevers in this area.

As chief investigator, Gordon plotted the unique, geographically circumscribed epidemiology of what was called coastal fever over the course of two wet seasons.

First wet season
Gordon initiated a far-ranging study that involved patients with symptoms of coastal fever, wild animals that they may have contacted, and epidemiological information to ascertain occupational and lifestyle exposure to insects and 'unhealthy' environments.

In Cairns, Gordon conducted clinical examinations and collected material from patients at the Cairns Base Hospital with symptoms of coastal fever who came from Mossman Gorge, about 60 kilometres north of Cairns, to Tully, 120 kilometres south. Most of these patients lived or worked in scrubland in the mountain range along the coastal belt.

An agreement between the Queensland Department of Health and the IMVS provided a supply of a specific species of white mice that was susceptible to the growth of intracellular bacteria that could not be grown on artificial culture media. These mice were transported to Cairns in batches for inoculation with specimens from patients and studies on the pathogenicity (disease-causing capability) of any microorganisms isolated from patient material. During his research, some infected mice were sent down to Adelaide for detailed study at the IMVS. The South Australian Museum and The University of Adelaide had expert entomologists and parasite specialists who reviewed material sent down by Gordon.

The study groups were:

1. An initial 15 patients, one of whom had typhus confirmed by a high titre in the Weil Felix agglutination test, and white mice who became ill after inoculation with patient blood. Three mice that demonstrated fever and symptoms consistent with typhus infection were sent back to the IMVS in Adelaide for confirmation that the mice were ill with typhus.
   The remaining 14 patients demonstrated anthrax-like bacilli in their clotted blood that was observed microscopically before inoculation into mice and being introduced to a range of artificial media incubated at 37°C.
2. 70 rats and 7 bandicoots – wild caught.
3. A further 40 febrile patients underwent venesection and their clotted blood was incubated at 'room' temperature (23°C). The incubating culture media were inspected microscopically every few days using a *Rickettsia*-specific stain (Laigret and Auburtin).

The findings from the first year of study were published in the *Medical Journal of Australia*.

1. It has been shown that (classical) cases of typhus comprise only a small percentage of the previously undiagnosed fevers of North Queensland.
2. After other known conditions have been separated, the residue of the cases of coastal fever appear to constitute a single disease entity.

3. Transmission appears to be by a vector, which may be a mite, mosquito or tick.
4. From the patients presenting with the symptoms listed above, an organism that is a member of the anthrax group has invariably been isolated. This organism appears to be the causal agent of the disease, but it is also found in the blood in cases of typhus. It is present in 70% of captured rats and bandicoots.
5. The organism is pleomorphic and is usually seen as a Gram-negative bacillus with bi-polar staining, or a Gram-positive anthrax-like bacillus. It grows readily on or in artificial media at 20–30°C but will not multiply appreciatively at 37°C when the media are directly inoculated with a patient's blood.

This first report into coastal fever produced some unexpected results, the most surprising being the presence of anthrax-like bacilli in the blood of febrile patients and from wild bandicoots and rats.

The experimental protocol had been established with a view to finding bacteria of the typhus type that only grow in experimental animals like mice. Multiple attempts to grow bacteria on artificial media from patients with symptoms of typhus failed in the hands of numerous investigators. The fact that Gordon Heaslip managed to culture bacteria on artificial media from the blood of patients with symptoms of typhus is *a priori* evidence that those bacteria were responsible for the patient's symptoms. This conclusion is reinforced by the fact that when the anthrax-like bacteria are inoculated into experimental animals they cause a disease that is identical to experimental typhus. At autopsy the tissue pathology in mice demonstrates intracellular infection and systemic disease consistent with typhus.

A further unexpected result was that the anthrax-like bacillus grew preferentially at 22°C rather than 37°C; pathogenic (disease-causing) bacteria generally grow at body temperature (37°C), while saprophytic (environmental and harmless) bacteria grow preferentially at 22°C.

Gordon considered the possibility of contaminants and took special care when he inoculated a range of media and animals with patient samples. However, the consistency of the results from patients both microscopically and on culture reinforced the conclusion that these bacteria were the cause of coastal fever. Gordon believed that he had found a new microbial cause for coastal fever, not a contaminant. He arranged further experiments to take account of the findings that this bacillus grew preferentially at 22°C.

Major change of direction
The search for causes of fevers in North Queensland started on the premise that the likely cause was a microorganism that could not be grown on artificial media and was probably a species of typhus unique to North Queensland. The finding of a bacterium that grew on artificial media from patients with fever and symptoms of coastal completely changed the focus of the study.

The anthrax-like bacillus was certainly not a *Rickettsia*, but the dilemma for Gordon was that these bacilli were found in patients with symptoms of typhus and a positive Weil Felix agglutination test (the diagnostic test for typhus which detects antibodies that recognise specific proteus bacteria (OXK, O19 strains) associated with epidemic typhus – the most serious form of typhus). Gordon's findings immediately raised doubts that at least some fevers in North Queensland were not typhus, as was previously assumed.

What was the role of this unexpected bacterium that seemed to be closely associated with the fevers in North Queensland? At this point, Gordon continued with his research on the hypothesis that there may be two causes for fevers in North Queensland, namely febrile patients infected with the anthrax-like bacteria and those with typhus.

The next phase of investigation concentrated on patients who definitely had typhus according to the criteria used at the time, which was a clinical history of fever, sometimes rash, an eschar signifying the 'entry' vector bite, and a positive Weil Felix agglutination test. These patients were then compared with patients infected with the anthrax-like bacillus associated with their fever.

At this point, Gordon considered that coastal fever might be a specific disease associated with the anthrax-like bacillus and that typhus was a separate infection. He also considered that possibility of a 'double' infection with both microorganisms. He reported the overall clinical and laboratory findings in his second publication 'Tsutsugamushi Fever in North Queensland, Australia' (*Medical Journey of Australia*, 29 March 1941). This second publication built upon observations in his first report, and is regarded as Gordon Heaslip's definitive paper on fevers in North Queensland. The paper lists all 54 patients who fulfilled the definition of typhus associated with Tsutsugamushi fever that had been observed in North Queensland previously and was widespread in the Asian region.

The results were presented in a series of tables that provided the data upon which the diagnosis of typhus was determined. The investigations undertaken on each patient are tabulated over five pages.

Certain investigations in some patients were listed as N.U. (not used), N.D. (no data), and N.S. (not seen). In discussion Gordon indicated that subjects with missing data were included as cases of typhus if they were epidemiologically associated with other cases and other investigations, for example if the agglutination of Proteus titre was highly positive for typhus.

Gordon's comments on these results are surprising because he scarcely mentions the major findings in the first report, which described the presence of a new species of bacterium that had never been described in association with any fever or illness. This second report was confined to patients who had clinical evidence of typhus, however most patients with typhus were also infected with the anthrax-like bacillus described in his first report.

In essence, these results were inconclusive in terms of determining the exact cause of coastal fever. The experimental results were not subjected to statistical analysis and the role of the anthrax-like bacillus was conjectural. Nevertheless, Gordon undertook further laboratory studies to confirm its classification.

Research in Cairns ceases

The IMVS had begun providing laboratory supplies and training to military hospitals throughout Australia. Gordon was an expert on agglutination and bacteriology tests, which were important investigations to distinguish the causes of fever in the tropics such as malaria, dengue and typhus, so that appropriate management of the patient could be provided.

In 1939, at the conclusion of these clinical investigations in Cairns, Gordon returned to the IMVS to complete laboratory research on this new strain of bacterium, which he named microorganism *Bacillus tropicus*. He brought several specimens of the anthrax-like bacillus to the IMVS where he completed detailed laboratory analysis to conclude that this bacterium was a new species associated with coastal fever. Gordon wrote:

> *The preliminary part of this work was performed at the Commonwealth Health Laboratory at Cairns, North Queensland. Subsequently various strains were more fully investigated in Adelaide, and the results form the basis of this paper. The work was prematurely terminated on account of military service.*

Detailed laboratory studies were performed according to the requirements specified in D.H. Bergey's *Manual of Determinative Bacteriology*. The results of the various tests led Gordon to conclude that the anthrax-like bacillus associated with fevers in North Queensland was a member of the genus *Bacillus* belonging to Group A, 1 of Division I in the Bergey classification (1939), page 697.

In the publication Gordon states:

> *The grounds on which* Bacillus tropicus *has been designated as a new species are the cultural peculiarities and the common occurrence in man and animals in the coastal region of North Queensland, and possibly elsewhere. Owing to the apparent restriction of the organism to the tropics and to the fact that it was isolated in the tropical portion of Australia, it has been named* Bacillus tropicus.

> *Cultures have been deposited in the Laboratory of Pathology and Microbiology, Brisbane, and the Institute of Medical and Veterinary Science, Adelaide, and sent to the United States Department of Agriculture, Washington, D.C.*

The results of his research at IMVS were published in the *Medical Journal of Australia* in 1941. Following this publication, Gordon never returned to medical research.

NHMRC research in North Queensland

Gordon's key findings published after the entirety of his research:

- People with coastal fever in the Cairns area were infected with a hitherto unknown bacterium which Gordon named *Bacillus tropicus*. *Bacillus tropicus* was cited in Topley and Wilson's *Principles of Bacteriology and Immunity*, the international authority on bacterial infections. Several research reports outlined the association of anthrax-like bacteria with various diseases. The entry in Topley and Wison indicates that *B tropicus* was isolated from patients with tropical disease.
- Patients with scrub typhus in the Cairns area were also infected with *B tropicus*.
- Patients with coastal fever and/or typhus reported insect bites in association with their fevers. Epidemiology demonstrated that the people who developed fever had been associated with native bush and come into contact with trombiculid chiggers (larvae of mites) in the course of their occupation as timber workers, surveyors or others living adjacent to bushlands.
- 2500 specimens of larval trombids from 200 captured animals in the environs of infected humans were sent to colleagues in Adelaide for identification.
- *Trombicula deliensis* was suspected as the species of trombid most likely to have been the vector for transmitting fever (either typhus or coastal fever) from native animals to humans.

In the early stages of the war, Gordon served in the Citizen Military Forces while teaching nurses to be laboratory technicians and tutoring medical pathologists in the laboratory systems being supported by the IMVS.

Gordon enlisted in the full-time Australian Army Medical Corps (AAMC) at Wayville, Adelaide, on 23 June 1941. He was initially posted to military hospitals around Australia, and later posted in Morotai, Borneo at the conclusion of the war.

These findings of his research in Queensland and Adelaide were not published until Gordon was full-time as a pathologist in military hospitals. Most likely he was unaware of their publication and the impact that his research findings might have had on science in general or the understanding of tropical fevers.

Importance and impact of Gordon's research in North Queensland
The US Army had encountered problems of fevers and itch mites in PNG and the Pacific theatres of war. They cited Heaslip's papers in planning their management of these maladies among the troops. The most helpful information was the description of the larva and the first aid treatment that was applied to prevent progression onto fever and disability.

In Adelaide, Herbert Womersley diligently inspected the ticks and mites sent by Gordon and identified various new species of *Trombicula*. He published this finding in association with Gordon in 1943 (H. Womersley, A.L.S., F.R.E.S., South Australian Museum, and W.G. Heaslip M.B.B.S., 'The Trombiculae (Acarina) or Itch-Mites of the Austro-Malayan and Oriental Regions', *Trans. Roy. Society of South Australia*, 67, (1), 30 July 1943). This publication identified the limited number of species of trombiculids that were present in environmental fauna that transmitted infections to humans. Included in this publication is the recognition of Gordon's diligent research and collection of mites and ticks by naming the species *Trombicula fletcheri Womersley and Heaslip* 1943 as a vector of Tsutsugamushi disease (scrub typhus) in New Guinea.

Gordon was convinced that *B. tropicus*, the anthrax-like bacillus he identified as the cause for coastal fever, was a major scientific discovery. When he identified the anthrax-like bacillus he regarded it as the cause for significant disease. Several research reports in the *Journal of Infectious Diseases* and the *Journal of Clinical Pathology* published in the wake of Gordon's research have outlined the association of anthrax-like bacteria with various diseases.

An intriguing aspect of Gordon's meticulous bacteriological observations was that *B. tropicus* and *Rickettsia* bacteria were both present in people with symptoms of coastal fever and typhus.

Gordon was not alone in this observation, and he recognised the work of Ludwick Anigstein, an international expert on vector-borne diseases who had been studying epidemic typhus in Hungary and was a UN consultant on vector-borne diseases. Anigstein was recruited to study tropical fevers in Malaya. He reported a similar bacterium with similar characteristics as *B. tropicus*: it grew at room temperature and underwent changes in appearance and properties upon subculture. Despite these similarities, Anigstein contended that it was a form of typhus and called it *Rickettsia tropicalis*.

Gordon was aware of Anigstein's findings and wrote in his discussion for the *Medical Journal of Australia* March 1941 paper:

> 4. There is little doubt that some of the organisms isolated by Anigstein (1933) in Malaya were identical with mine, and he carried out experiments with human volunteers. In this way he succeeded in producing fever which was very similar to coastal fever, and which was, in some cases, almost certainly not typhus as he supposed.

The reports from Gordon's research and the work of Anigstein were published at the commencement of WWII. Neither Gordon nor Anigstein returned to follow up on their research on this typhus-like condition: Gordon was unable to continue because he was discharged from the army with a chronic disease, and Anigstein because he emigrated to the USA under the patronage of the Jewish Emigré

Committee in New York and gained a permanent research position at the University of Texas Medical Branch at Galveston where he turned his attention to antibiotics.

Gordon's war

After a pathology course in Eastern Command, Gordon returned to Fort Largs on 20 August 1941 and was then sent to Alice Springs on 1 October 1941. He was next attached to 10 Casualty Clearing Station (CCS) and sent to Darwin on 24 April 1942, where he was pathologist at the 119 Australian General Hospital, which had been transferred to Adelaide River after the Japanese bombing of Darwin on 19 February 1942.

On 1 September 1942 Gordon was promoted to the rank of major and served at 116 Australian General Hospital in Charters Towers. This hospital was established on the racecourse and the Mount Carmel College was requisitioned to accommodate nursing staff. Gordon returned to Adelaide between postings at various military general hospitals.

In October 1944 he joined the 2/14th Australian General Hospital in Townsville, and on 9 August 1945 he transferred to 2/5 Australian General Hospital at Morotai, Borneo. He served with 1 Papua New Guinea recruit unit before being posted to 9 Prisoner of War Recovery Group immediately after peace had been declared in the Pacific.

On 9 September 1945, Gordon commenced duties on Morotai. This island in Indonesia contained the main frontline combat formation of the RAAF in 1944–45. It was a major command post for the war in the Pacific and was utilised immediately after the war as a staging post for the return of prisoners of war. Gordon continued service with the AIF as a pathologist in the medical facilities where the Australian Prisoners of War (POW) were hospitalised while receiving care and rehabilitation; most were emaciated, suffering from parasite infestations and in need of nutrition and care for the ulcers and injuries sustained over months to years of deprivation.

While in Morotai, Gordon suffered from an acute episode of haematemesis and melaena (bleeding) thought to be caused by a duodenal ulcer. He was flown to Labuan and embarked USAT *Georgetown Victory,* arriving in Brisbane on 4 February 1946. After arriving in Brisbane, he was assessed and transferred to Adelaide's Daw Park Military Hospital on 27 February, where he underwent various diagnostic procedures. The investigations for the bleeding duodenal ulcer revealed that Gordon had a very high haemoglobin concentration, despite losing blood in recent weeks. Further tests indicated that he had an underlying condition that was a known to cause bleeding from ulcers, namely polycythaemia vera. This is a chronic condition caused by excessive production of red blood cells from the bone marrow.

After his condition stabilised, he was transferred to Kapara, a convalescent home on 25 March. On 1 April he underwent final assessment at Daw Park where final preparations were made for ongoing care in the community. Accordingly, he was 'Medical Boarded at 105' (assessed by the Military Medical Board) and declared unfit for duty 'due to duodenal ulcer and Polycythaemia (Rubra) Vera (negligible)'. He was formally discharged from the military on 8 April 1946.

Gordon's PCV condition was regarded as a genetic condition that was not associated with his military duties. Accordingly, he was not eligible for care by the Department of Veterans Affairs.

Life after the war for Gordon was a return to his early life in agriculture.

Chapter 6

Farming, Family, National Health

While recuperating from complications of polycythaemia vera [PCV] in Daw Park Hospital and Kapara Red Cross Rehabilitation Centre in Glenelg, Gordon contemplated his future.

He knew he could pursue an active life for at least 10 to 15 years providing he undertook regular blood tests and underwent venesection [phlebotomy] at the Red Cross transfusion centre every few months to maintain normal levels of red blood cells.

Gordon established his office in the large family home at Park Road, Kensington Park, replete with orchard, towering eucalypts and a tennis court. There was room for the offspring to roam as schoolchildren and young teenagers, and space for Barbara to pursue her community interests.

With boundless energy to achieve in his remaining life, Gordon set about creating two new major agricultural developments.

The first was a family-owned sheep station called Gilles Downs, a pastoral lease south-west of Iron Knob in South Australia. Over recent years the property had deteriorated due to drought and family interest in other properties in the Mid North.

The second was in the Ninety Mile Desert around Coonalpyn in the Southeast of the state, where the South Australian Government was remediating nutrient-deficient Crown land. Special provision was made for returned soldiers with farming experience to develop large tracts of this land into arable farms at small cost per acre. Gordon established the Dayspring Development Company to undertake this venture.

Both Gilles Downs and the Coonalpyn land holdings were poorly developed properties requiring fencing, clearing, sinking of dams, establishment of accommodation and preparation for stocking and cropping.

Gordon was hands on with planning and supervision of works on-site involving family and contractors using the most modern machinery and farming techniques. This suited Gordon's early farming experience and scientific/medical knowledge to create profitable farmland in the Heaslip tradition.

Life for Gordon after the war was divided between family, office and health care in Adelaide, and managing his agricultural properties in Gilles Downs where he was remediating a run-down station, and in Coonalpyn where he was establishing a new farm in rejuvenated scrub in the 90-mile desert.

Family

The children were able to attend schools within easy reach of their Kensington Park home and Barbara spent time with community causes, in particular meeting up with Doris Taylor who was politically active in supporting the Labor Party and causes for social justice. Barbara acted as chauffer for Doris Taylor, who was wheelchair bound after childhood injuries and a beguiling raconteur and general mover and shaker for social causes, including the establishment of Meals on Wheels.

Gordon was often supervising works at Gilles Downs and Dayspring Development. In Adelaide he had to check his health status and attend Red Cross for phlebotomy. Increasingly he became involved with government and land development authorities and committees. But family life very much revolved around Barbara.

Barbara and Gordon's eldest daughter Jocelyn wrote *Adelaide Woman*, a book that described life at home when Gordon was travelling extensively, and the community activities that Barbara supported. Jocelyn often accompanied Gordon on driving trips to Coonalpyn and business trips.

Barbara Shorney

The following extracts from *Adelaide Woman* and commentary about Barbara are provided by Jocelyn's son, Peter Preece.

Barbara was born into a well-to-do church family at Hall Street, Semaphore, a seaside suburb of Adelaide, in 1907, the youngest of four children. They were a talented and well-educated family, with Barbara and her sister Margaret both dux of Adelaide's Methodist Ladies College, and all three of the girls, including Winifred, attending the University of Adelaide, with Margaret studying medicine.

But tragedy haunted Barbara; by 1915 her sister Margaret had died of meningitis and her beloved brother was killed in action at Gallipoli. During the whole of her life Barbara found ANZAC Day an ordeal. In 1919, Barbara's father and grandmother died, and around the same time her sister Winifred had developed a brain tumour requiring surgery that left her with life-long disabilities.

Barbara excelled at her studies and started at university in 1925 aged 18 years. Here she met Gordon, aged 23 and in his second year of medical studies. By 1926 both were active in university student affairs, including the Christian Union and League of Nations Club, and in October of the following year were engaged to be married. It seems neither family thought they were a good match, having very little in common, and both thought them too young. Barbara was 20 years old.

Barbara graduated from the University of Adelaide in 1928, the first female in her family to do so, and soon after embarked on a world trip with her mother and surviving sister Winifred. This long trip, ostensibly to visit relatives in America and Europe, may have been contrived by Barbara's mother to temporarily separate Barbara and Gordon. After a few months away tragedy struck again with the sudden death in Canada of Barbara's mother. The trip was cut short, and the orphaned girls returned to Adelaide to bury their mother. Barbara and Gordon were married a fortnight later.

Early the following year, 1930, Gordon and Barbara moved to Sydney for six months while Gordon undertook a course of study for missionaries preparing to work in the Pacific islands. In September of that year they returned to Adelaide briefly before embarking for Papua New Guinea, and four years at the newly constructed missionary hospital at Salamo, Fergusson Island. In the book *Adelaide Woman* the author mentions the local pythons and crocodiles, pay-back killings, un-Christian-like sexual practices and cannibalism, and wonders how Barbara viewed these practices given that her upbringing had sheltered her from everything but the most polite human interactions.

Indeed, these must have been very trying times. According to *Adelaide Woman*:

> *there's no doubt that five long years living in such a demanding environment were hard on these two young people, and very hard on their relationship. The stoic Gordon, who had to battle serious problems of life and death, would, I believe, have eventually become impatient with Barbara's fears, and he may even have begun to speak harshly to her on occasion. The whole experience must have been an enormous test for them both. We know that by the end of it they had each lost their faith.*

In October 1935, Gordon resigned suddenly from his position managing the Solano missionary hospital and training centre and 'left with his family [now including two infants and an Adelaide nanny, Lorna Stacey] on the first boat'. The reason(s) don't appear to be clear, but a report cited in *Adelaide Woman* mentions 'ill-health', possibly 'a nervous breakdown of some sort'. From this time, it seems, 'Barbara and Gordon cut all ties with organised religion . . . and Gordon who had attended church every Sunday of his life until now, never did so again . . .'

At this stage life appears to be approaching a conventional normality of sorts:

> *On his return from New Guinea, Gordon had found employment as a pathologist with the Institute of Medical and Veterinary Science, and for a short time enjoyed a more relaxed home life with his young family, indulging himself with some backyard tomato growing, and playing tennis and golf.*

In mid-1937, Barbara and Gordon, leaving their young family in Adelaide in the care of Lorna the nanny, embarked on a nine-month world tour including the coronation of King George VI in London.

> *Towards the end of 1938, with war looming, the government asked Gordon to carry out research in tropical medicine in Cairns. Barbara, Lorna and the two children followed in January 1939, and they were there for almost two years. Something happened in Cairns that signalled the first hints of a serious breakdown in the marriage. Barbara accused Gordon of having been unfaithful.*
>
> *By September 1940, England had declared war on Germany, Gordon had resigned, and the family were back in Adelaide. Japan was suspected of preparing to invade the Philippines. Two months later, Gordon was appointed a Captain with the Australian Army Medical Corps Reserve.*

By now Barbara was expecting her third child and had purchased the much larger house in Kensington Park. Gordon was away for most of the war apart from occasional visits when in Australia, with Barbara left to manage the large house and the young family. This must have been a difficult time for many families, as described in *Adelaide Woman:*

> *The difficulties facing couples whose domestic roles had been fractured by years of war service were epic – the stuff of classic tragedy. Let's imagine the woman who's been shouldering all the family responsibility and making all the decisions for five or six years. She may have been raising children alone and may have had to face all sorts of problems, including serious childhood illnesses.*
>
> *Imagine her overnight having to adjust to someone else being in charge in her home; a virtual stranger who barely knows, let alone understands, her or her children. She may have been desperately lonely in his absence, while he may have become used to the camaraderie of the 'mess'.*
>
> *How could they possibly just resume their old lives as though nothing had changed?*

Gordon and Barbara's lives continued to diverge after the war. Gordon took up land development interests, including Gilles Downs Station, via Iron Knob, grazing via Tintinara, and a residential subdivision in Parafield Gardens, South Australia.

Barbara pursued her own interests including action to improve the working conditions of nurses, the establishment of Meals on Wheels with her close friend Doris Taylor, advocating for the frail aged and the mentally ill. This involved petitions and numerous letters to politicians and the people of South Australia. She was also active in the peace movement, this latter interest attracting the attention of Australia's security police force, ASIO.

Barbara's physical and mental health suffered during this time and she experienced frequent bouts of depression, and a morphine addiction following major surgery.

In June 1954, Barbara was certified and sent to Enfield Receiving Home and as part of her treatment was given electroconvulsive, or 'shock' therapy. It was here that she met skilled and passionate people in whose care her health improved. She began to make many changes to practices and procedures from within the hospital and even requested a longer stay. She was instrumental in establishing Alcoholics Anonymous in South Australia and the South Australian State Commission on Alcoholism, and went on to write several books on mental health and had a wing at Hillcrest Hospital named after.

Barbara Kate Heaslip died in 1982 in her sleep at home in Mitcham, South Australia.

Gordon's medical career

After the war, when Gordon chose to cease practising medicine, there was no sadness because he felt that his medical career was dominantly in laboratory medicine and research. In these phases of his career, he made important contributions to the war effort and his discoveries about the *Trombicula deliensis* mite being the vector for transmitting scrub typhus to humans resulted in new understandings about the ecology and natural history of Trombiculid mites worldwide.

As a medical practitioner he felt that he lacked rapport with patients. When his daughter Rosalie asked him why he did not stay a doctor, he answered that he did not have the bedside manner to be a good doctor.

Reflecting on his medical education and career as a medical missionary, pathologist and medical researcher Gordon felt strongly that the medical profession should be practising preventive medicine alongside treatments for disease, and that the key to improving national health was through improvements in medical education.

Gordon published an article* that summarised his views about how community health would be best served. In essence, he felt that his own medical education was deficient in preparing graduates to pursue strategies that would prevent disease in the community. He believed the course prepared graduates to treat diseases and become 'specialist' medical practitioners and that the medical training should be revised to prepare graduates to improve health outcomes of the community.

This milestone article differs from his past research reports, which predominantly focused on the area of insect-borne fevers, with some commentary about the polio epidemic that occurred on his watch when he was with the IMVS. But why did Gordon choose to comment on the direction of national health in Australia?

This was a time when the Australian postwar government was considering something akin to the British National Health scheme. The following extracts from his article 'National Health' give a strong indication of Gordon's abiding interest in how best to achieve a national health system for Australia.

> *The untimely dead sent to their graves by preventable accident or disease, the inmates of hospitals and institutions who suffer needlessly through ignorance and poverty, and the deformed and disabled, so many of whom are living memorials to ineptitude, all bear witness to the imperfection of our national health and to the inadequacy of our health service.*

---

*   W.G. Heaslip, 'National Health', *Medical Journal of Australia*, 6 July 1946

The medical profession cannot of itself supply what is required to bring optimal health.

The war has shown, particularly in Britain, that the public health may improve dramatically when the number of medical practitioners has been drastically reduced, and the remainder are working under difficult circumstances.

While it is well that members [of the medical profession] should remember that their profession originated from witchcraft and superstition, it is high time they realised that they are public servants and not high priests.

The provision of an adequate curative service, with some attempts at prevention is not enough. What is required is that an adequate curative be made available to everyone irrespective of their position geographically, financially, or morally, and that provision be implemented to the limit of available knowledge. It is becoming obvious that health is much more dependent on social structure than on medical practice, and that education is more important than medication.

*It cannot be very long before the profession will be asked why it remains satisfied with attempting to cure disease which it should have prevented. It may well be accused openly that (*inter alia) *it is failing: to educate and train its members adequately.*

For a great many years, the sick in mind, as well as the sick in body have been given infusions instead of instruction, and pills instead of propaganda.

Every medical student should be taught that: (a) each disability should be investigated from the aspect of prevention as well as correction; (b) every endeavour and resource should be used to discover the causes of an illness or accident; (c) not only the primary, but also the contributing causes, should be discovered and removed.

The complete *Medical Journal of Australia* article is provided as an appendix.

The existing separation between research workers and clinicians must be removed so that there may be maximum use of clinical data, maximum applications of research findings, and a more intelligent and orderly direction of research.

Gordon remained registered as a medical practitioner and undertook occasional locum-tenens duties for friends, but devoted most of his time to agriculture and family matters.

To achieve his aspirations to improve national health outcomes through medical education and preventive health, Gordon made a bequest for medical education and preventive health when he developed terminal complications of his PCV.

Chapter 7

Gordon's Last Years: Agriculture and a Bequest

Gordon knew his condition of polycythemia vera would progress after 15 years of relatively healthy life. Throughout this time, his life became frenetic. He supported his family financially and visited home to maintain health treatments and attend to business affairs. The distance grew between Gordon and his wife Barbara, who was obsessively focused on different activities.

Agriculture and land development
Gilles Downs was purchased for £4300 in 1924 by Gordon's father as a pastoral lease. Fencing was laid and a dam built to support stock. It remained largely undeveloped until Gordon purchased it in August 1946 for £18,000 and immediately set about improving fencing and housing and stocking it with sheep who thrived on the plentiful saltbush in the area.

It took several years of Gordon's supervision of on-site workers to bring the property up to a productive sheep station.

A further opportunity for acquiring farming land arose when the South Australian Government decided to remediate large tracts of Crown land that was unproductive. Early attempts using European farming techniques on this Mallee scrub failed to conserve moisture and promoted sand drift. Water-borne soil and wind erosion leeched nutrients from the stony and sandy soil. Research by the Department of Agriculture, CSIRO, and Waite Institute indicated that these soils were unable to conserve water and were deficient in essential nutrients. Experimental farms established that these sandy soils could become productive by the addition of trace elements copper and zinc to superphosphate fertiliser, and planting certain strains of clover to improve soil structure.

After the war, large tracts of land were remediated and made available for new farm development. The largest area was 160,000 hectares in the Upper Southeast known as the Ninety Mile Desert. This was the last major land development in South Australia and arrangements were made for private consortiums to tender for remediation and development of the land for agricultural use.

The major developer was the Australian Mutual Provident Society [AMP] who financed the overall remediation. The clearing of bush in the late 1940s was achieved on a large scale with powerful D7 tractors hauling huge logs to knock down the larger trees, followed by a heavy anchor chain dragged between two tractors to level the soil for remediation with trace elements and cropping. After initial clearing and provision of access roads and infrastructure large allotments were sold for further development by landowners

In South Australia, the *War Service Land Settlement Act 1945*, passed on 3 January 1946, enabled WWII veterans to purchase land at reduced prices to take up farming with support from the State and Commonwealth Government. Gordon Heaslip purchased a large parcel of this land west of Tintinara at 2/6 per acre and created the Dayspring Development Company.

Dayspring Development Company

The Dayspring Development Company took up one large allotment and subdivided it into a series of subdivisions for cropping and grazing. This occurred over several years, commencing with the clearing of the scrub, preparing the soil, establishing roads and planning community centres. The town of Tintinara was the focus for local government and community centres, which occupied the site of a homestead established by graziers who moved into the area in the 1840s with large flocks of sheep.

Gordon Heaslip was actively involved in Government committees with oversight of the development. He became a member of the Coonalpyn District Council, joined the Stockowner's Association of South Australia (where he progressed to the executive and ultimately treasurer for three years prior to his death). Rosalie wrote:

> *He seemed to be responsible for the building of the Tintinara Hotel, perhaps in the capacity as District Councillor. I am sure he had shares in the Hotel, as I remember him growling about the power bill and that the fact that one light switch would turn on several lights when only one light was necessary.*

When all the blocks had been prepared for establishing separate farms Gordon chose one for the family development and sold the others. By early 1950s he was devoting much time to developing Dayspring as a cropping and grazing farm. A homestead had been established and his son Jeffrey was working on the farm to complete the clearing and establish the crops.

Jeffrey Heaslip's recollection

My first recollection of Dayspring was camping in a patch of low heath and mallee with my father and his youngest brother, Lloyd, in 1947, not far from an old shepherd's hut inhabited by bees, one of my enduring memories.

Dad's idea was to provide ex-servicemen with a 1000-acre block of land for which they worked for three years and bought at cost. The only people I can remember doing so are Jim Bourne and his family, who moved farther south-east after a short time; Reg Dow, with whom I lived for a year; and Arthur and Joyce Hannaford and their children, who were the only successful (if that is the appropriate word) members of the scheme.

Jim lived in the shed at the north-east corner of the property while the house on top of the hill to the south was being built, and then for a time in the house. The only other inhabitant of the shed was Lofty Morris, who worked for Dad on Gilles Downs, 13 miles south-west of

Iron Knob, prior to his time on Dayspring. I have no idea how long he spent there but I did see him one day in 1965 outside the Gresham Hotel on the corner of King William Street and North Terrace. We sat in the gutter and had a yarn. He was working somewhere in the Snowy Mountains.

I began working for my father early in 1954 after Jim had left and when Arthur and Joyce were in the stone place. I left at the end of 1959, after spending most of my time picking stones and stumps, carting and spreading hundreds of tons of superphosphate (a bag an acre every year), digging wells, erecting windmills and installing troughs, putting up miles of fencing (the last one of which is still there on the south side of the road opposite Arthur's place), crushing stone for the more sandy patches of the tracks, and the other bits and pieces common to all farms.

We ran a large flock of merino ewes, which were mated to Romney Marsh rams to produce a top quality fat lamb for the English market (£4 a head when our wage was £10 a week). We also ran a herd of about 50 cows mated with Aberdeen Angus bulls and used two stock horses. One was a mare that was well broken and no trouble to catch but had no idea of what she was doing. Keeping her under control was a full-time job. Let the reins go slack for an instant and she was off, straight through the middle of the mob. On one occasion, on the way back to unsaddle, I let her have her head in the paddock behind the shearer's quarters. At the gate into the holding paddock she wanted to turn in while I wanted to continue the ride. She hit the strainer post with an almighty thump and took it clean out of the ground, all three feet of it. She went one way and the post and I went the other. I don't know what she felt like the next morning, but I could hardly move. The old gelding was the quietest thing on four legs you could ever wish to ride. You could doze off in the saddle while he kept the mob in order and was wonderful at cutting out cattle from the mob. His only drawback was that he was 17 hands high. Fortunately I'd been a good gymnast at school, and pretty agile, so I didn't have to use a ladder. I mention this only because of my height: five feet and half an inch.

Early in the scheme of things, Dad bought a property on the eastern side of Murray Bridge. He installed Lawrie Cockshell, from Jaybuk, as a mechanic (his son, John still lives at Tailem Bend) and grew oranges. A pump was installed several feet above the highest previously recorded flood but that didn't stop the 1956 flood rising two feet above the pumphouse.

When Arthur and Joyce moved to the house on their own property, I moved to the stone house and lived in the room at the end of the garage in the backyard. My housekeepers and working men were Tom and Eileen Lawless, followed by Kevin and Judy Clark and, somewhere in there, Bob Lampe who stayed only a year or so. After a couple of years, I moved to the shearers' quarters and was still living there when I left. For periodic company I had Jack Briggs from Melrose with his shearers (and sons) for crutching and shearing twice a year; a young English lad for a while, Terry Kirby, and two big strong German boys, Otto the wiry one, and Eric the burly one, who put the flooring in the woolshed. They showed me how to get a bag of super under each arm and carry them on to the truck instead of using a sack truck. I preferred the sack truck. There were also a couple of surveyors who surveyed the western part beyond Hannaford's. My longest surviving housemate was Frank Brock, one of the easiest blokes to get on with I have ever met.

Water was always a problem, which explains why the country was called Ninety Mile Desert. We only solved it by digging wells, which ranged in depth from about 10 feet to 20. Bores proved useless and were responsible for two episodes that I would rather forget. The first was that I dropped a perfectly good hammer down one. The second was that I had to cut a length of bore-casing in two with a hacksaw. Try it sometime. The usable water sat on top of the unusable water such that if we went too deep, we had to back fill it until it was usable. The depth of usable water was two to three feet, but it varied a little. The wells were timbered with old sleepers, which we picked up on the railway line. We cut them to size with a circular saw, cut toggles and fitted them when the well was as deep as it could be. A mill, fitted with a sand screen, and a trough finished the job. Theoretically it was barely suitable for sheep, being about 1000 grains, but the stock got used to it. Our stock losses were much higher than would normally be tolerated, about 10%, but a lot of that was due to foxes and thieves.

Community service
Gordon travelled extensively from his home in Kensington Park to properties near Tintinara, Adelaide city, land at Parafield Gardens and the family station at Gilles Downs. He sold the vacant city land for a car park and subdivided the Parafield Gardens property into a housing estate, where he named the streets after the women in four generations of his family.

In his busy schedule he made time to participate in worthy causes, no doubt shaped by his family background in community service and philanthropy.

During his training as a missionary, he was a guest of Rev. John Wear Burton in Sydney, general secretary of the Methodist Missionary Society of Australasia. J.W. Burton had arranged for Gordon to complete a course in tropical medicine at the University of Sydney for six months before Gordon and Barbara embarked from Adelaide for Papua on 18 September 1930.

Burton was a life-long friend of Gordon's and an ardent pacifist, so it was not surprising that Gordon and Barbara embraced pacifism and became prominent in Adelaide as agitators for peace during the 1950s. This Cold War period included the Korean War, 1950–53, that involved Australian troops. The Communist Party of Australia was perceived as a threat by governments, and atomic tests were conducted by the British Government in Australia between 1953 and 1956.

Barbara and Gordon came to the attention of ASIO during this period when they hired community halls on occasion to accommodate pacifist meetings. Barbara's friend Doris Taylor was a determined fighter for social justice. She was secretary of the West Norwood sub branch of the Australian Labor Party, public relations officer in SA for the Australian Pensioners League, and campaigned strongly for the aged and infirm through political agitation, especially for the elderly.

Barbara Heaslip has a 'nervous breakdown', 1954

In the early 1950s, Barbara required major surgery and became overwhelmed to the point of decompensation. Barbara described this period in her life in her publication *Saints in Strait Jackets*.

> *I was certified in June 1954 and sent to Enfield Receiving Home.*
>
> *The precipitating cause of my brief attack was the refusal of Thomas Playford – later knighted – premier of South Australia, to accept a petition for a desperately needed infirmary for the aged, collected and paid for by me, urged on by my close friend, the late Doris Taylor OBE, founder of Meals on Wheels in South Australia. This petition of some 18,000 signatures had been signed by many members of the Establishment. But there had been a hiatus in time between its collection and its presentation due to surgery I had undergone, from which I almost died.*
>
> *I rushed to the* News, *declaiming that democracy was dead in South Australia, as indeed it was, as was to be for years to come, and that I would fly my petition to the Queen. Instead, I went to Enfield.*

Barbara was admitted to Enfield and then transferred to the Northfield Psychiatric Hospital, where she received therapy for a year. During this time, she came to understand the problems of patients with mental illnesses and the often-inhumane treatment they received. The year that Barbara was released from hospital, the drug Largactil became available for treating people with uncontrollable psychiatric diagnoses. The use of Largactil allowed large numbers of these patients to be released into the community.

Barbara continued to attend at Northfield for therapy sessions where she demonstrated care and compassion for her previous fellow patients, and during these times she came to work with Medical Superintendent

Dr William Salter to guide former patients in their return to life outside hospital. Many patients were in psychiatric hospitals because of alcohol excess and Dr Salter decided to tackle this community problem by starting a branch of Alcoholics Anonymous in South Australia.

Barbara Heaslip enjoyed her roles in helping psychiatric patients prepare for life 'outside hospital walls' and felt fulfilled. She was also a good public speaker with demonstrated skills in organising community gatherings.

From the late 1950s Barbara volunteered full-time for Northfield Hospital and Alcoholics Anonymous. She purchased several houses in the community for previous psychiatric patients and promoted AA at meetings around country regions.

The contribution of Barbara Heaslip to mental health was prodigious and long lasting. When a new extension was built at the Northfield Psychiatric Hospital it was named the Barbara Heaslip Wing.

Acute myeloid leukemia complicates polycythaemia

Polycythaemia vera was regarded as a benign condition that occurred in mid to later life and was manageable with regular venesections [removal of blood] to remove the excess red blood cells. Venesection diminishes the engorgement of veins, prevents thrombosis, ameliorates enlargement of the spleen, and reduces the cyanotic appearance that gave rise to the disease description polycythaemia rubra vera.

The frequency of venesection is generally two and three times per year, and the amount of blood removed is determined by the level of haemoglobin and haematocrit. Notwithstanding the inconvenience of regular venesection, a person with polycythaemia vera could maintain a normal life until the condition transforms from a benign production of excess red blood cells into a cancer that involved the bone marrow.

During 1960 Gordon's haematocrit was increasing, requiring more frequent venesection. Nevertheless, Gordon maintained his commercial interests and attended to his duties as treasurer of the Stockowners Association of South Australia, and Coonalpyn District Council.

In early 1961 he decided to sell his large property in Kensington Park. The property at 27 Park Road had been on the market for some months and he was having difficulty maintaining his multiple interests, so the property was sold to a developer who subsequently converted the main house into three flats and built four houses on the tennis court and orchard.

After selling the Kensington Park house, Gordon and Rosalie moved into a 'halfway house' at Blair Athol that Barbara had purchased, and he took rooms at his sister's house where he maintained his office.

In the frenzy of selling the house, relocating accommodation and tending to business affairs, Gordon's polycythaemia gene mutated and provoked a massive production of aggressive malignant cells from the bone marrow manifesting as myeloid leukaemia.

The first signs of leukaemia were fever and oedema of the skin as the leukemic cells filled the blood stream. Gordon was admitted to Royal Adelaide Hospital with shortness of breath as the lung was infiltrated with malignant cells causing a massive pneumonia. Over the next few days leukemic cells and excess fluid were removed from the blood stream and lungs.

This unexpected rapid deterioration left no time for Gordon to tidy up his business or family affairs. When he was admitted to hospital, Gordon's daughter Jennifer was alerted in England, and she arranged a flight return to Adelaide within 48 hours. This journey required eight stops and five days flying between London and Sydney. Gordon was barely alive when Jennifer arrived home in Adelaide just before his death.

Gordon had little time to finalise his affairs prior to his hospital admission. He had various joint-venture business arrangements, he had written scientific and medical articles that indicated his aspirations, and he had made his view known about matters he cared about. Gordon summoned his lawyers who prepared his last will and testament, finalised the day before his death on 27 October 1961 at Royal Adelaide Hospital.

The death certificate listed cause of death as 'Bronchial Pneumonia,

Myeloid Leukemia and Polycythaemia Vera 20 Years'. Gordon Heaslip was cremated on 30 October 1961.

In making his last will and testament, Gordon provided for his wife and family, and bequeathed funds to establish a Medical Education Trust Fund to fulfil his aspirations for medical education that he had expressed in the *Medical Journal of Australia* in 1946.

After Gordon's death
Barbara continued her community mental health support and enjoyed her role as grandmother to her many grandchildren.

Jeffrey finished school in 1951, then attended Roseworthy Agricultural College north of Gawler, graduating in 1954 along with many well-known individuals who progressed to the agriculture, viticulture and wine-making industries. From 1954 Jeff worked at Dayspring for five years before travelling extensively in the UK, Europe – including Eastern Europe – the Middle East and India. He attended the 1960 Rome Olympic Games. He returned to Australia and became a successful schoolteacher and principal in regional South Australia (including Iron Knob, not far from Gilles Downs and Port Lincoln). He married Marie Green and raised five children. In his retirement, Jeff's family established a successful vineyard, the Heaslip Winery in the Clare district.

Jocelyn completed her schooling at Girton Girls' School in Kensington Park in 1953. She moved to Billa Kalina Station in central South Australia as a governess to the Greenfield family during the Maralinga tests. She married and moved to Melbourne in 1955 where she had two of her four children. Gordon visited her in Melbourne at least once, during which time he caused an accident when his unattended Vanguard car rolled down a hill and smashed into neighbouring house in Montmorency, Melbourne.

Jocelyn and her family relocated to Adelaide in the early 1960s. She later trained in primary school education and had a successful career as a teacher in SA and later the Northern Territory. She had a close relationship with Gordon and regretted moving away to Melbourne for the last few years of his life.

Jenny went on to teachers' college after school and taught in various schools in regional South Australia as well as raising four children.

After Gordon's death, Rosalie became a nurse, raised four children and later settled in Geraldton, then Albany, Western Australia.

Chapter 8

Heaslip Bequest and Flinders School of Medicine

Agriculture, medicine, and health research dominated his professional life, and when it came to making his last will, Gordon chose to make a bequest to medical education as well as making provisions for his wife and family.

This chapter presents details of Gordon's bequest and an extended analysis of the uses to which it has been put, with recommendations for its future deployment for current Australian Health Reform.

Gordon bequeathed funds to establish a Medical Education Trust to be allocated to a single South Australian medical school selected by 'my Trustees to be used for the purpose of improving and keeping the education of medical undergraduates as modern and efficient as possible and in particular the training and education of graduates to qualify them in the principles and practice of teaching'.

When the bequest was made in 1961 there was only one medical school in South Australia at the University of Adelaide. Gordon would have been aware that provision was being made for a second university in the southern region, together with a public hospital and a second medical school to cater for the postwar population boom and industrial development in the south, which supported intensive agriculture, light industry, an oil refinery at Port Stanvac, and a Chrysler vehicle assembly plant at Tonsley.

In 1960, the State Government annexed 150 acres of Kaurna land at Bedford Park that had supported a sanatorium for soldiers with tuberculosis, and additional land that was set aside for a future teachers' college. A planning committee for the Bedford Park Campus of the University of Adelaide was established in 1961 with Professor Karmel as chair.

In 1965, students commenced studies in new buildings and the Labor State Government decided that the Bedford Park campus should become an independent second university in Adelaide, named after Matthew Flinders. The new campus was opened on 25 March by Her Majesty Queen Elizabeth, the Queen Mother. The *Flinders University Act* was enacted on 1 July 1966.

An academic medical centre to cater for health needs in the southern region was jointly established between Flinders University and the South Australian Health Department adjacent to the Flinders University. The inaugural Dean of the Flinders Medical School, Professor Gus Fraenkel, was appointed in 1970. The Flinders Medical Centre was built in time to enrol the first-year medical students in 1974. The teaching hospital began admitting students in 1976.

Allocation of the Heaslip Bequest
Gordon had achieved much in his agriculture endeavours, medical research, and community development. However, he was unable to influence his long-held aspiration of improving population health through medical education, outlined in his article published in the *Medical Journal of Australia* in 1946. The addition of the bequest in his will aimed to address the deficiencies he endured in his own medical education, and to improve health outcomes through medical education. The establishment of the bequest was delayed after Gordon's death in 1961 until the death of his wife Barbara on 10 May 1982.

Extracts of the Will of W.G. Heaslip
Gordon was very clear in his intention for the use of the bequest, outlining not only what the bequest was to be used for, but also why he felt the bequest was necessary in the first place.

[Clause 7] The selection of the South Australian medical school was to take into account the foregoing gifts:

(a) having suffered as a student at the hands of Professors and Lecturers who had been given no training as teachers and
(b) having seen the unfortunate results which may arise from the sectional teaching of medicine which should be taught as a whole and
(c) deploring the present tendency to produce a medical graduate who is a potential Specialist when he should be a General Practitioner and
(d) aware that there exists a continuing body of medical graduates who are desirous of improving and keeping high the standard of undergraduate medical education and
(e) believing that the achievement of this objective would be assisted by the provision of financial backing for suitable projects.

[Clause 8] In making this gift for the reasons set out above (which shall be borne in mind by the Trust Fund Trustees when considering an application for a grant until such reasons no longer have significance) I wish to impress upon the mind of the Trust Fund Trustees the fact that the practice of medicine has always had two inseparable aspects. One of these is the curative, which has been over emphasised in the past, the other is the preventative and this has been neglected. The medical undergraduate should have both these aspects as the basis for all his training, and it is my wish that the trust fund trustees will bear this in mind and emphasise it whenever an opportunity to do so presents itself.

[Clause 9] It is my wish that until the Trust Fund Trustees decide to make other of it the Trust Fund shall be made available to medical graduates who propose to proceed to or who are already engaged in the specialty of teaching to enable them to get instruction at an approved institution in the principles and practice of teaching.

Copies of the sections of the Will including Clause 14 are available on request to the Special Collection of the Flinders University Library together with correspondence between The Executor Trustee and Agency Company of South Australia and Jocelyn Preece.

The University of Adelaide or Flinders University?

The Executor Trustee and Agency Company of South Australia provided the information below in a letter to Jocelyn, Gordon's eldest daughter, dated 4 April 1985. She had requested clarification about why Flinders University Medical School was considered because it did not exist when the Will was written in 1961.

> *Clearly, therefore, Dr Heaslip foresaw the creation of, at the least, a second university in South Australia with a Medical Faculty. Had he not, the wording 'or such other South Australian University' appearing twice in Clause 14 would have been total unnecessary.*
>
> *As stated above, Clause 6 uses the singular 'a' and this is repeated in both instances in Clause 14.*
>
> *Accordingly, it is our belief that upon the true interpretation of the terms of the Trust, Dr Heaslip did intend that only one Medical School in South Australia should benefit. This being further reinforced by the wording in Clause 6 'to be selected by my Trustees' and again by the wording used initially in Clause 14 'my Trustees shall select' and later in the same Clause twice used 'as my Trustees shall select'.*
>
> *In accordance with the argument set out above the Trustees of the Estate must select either the University of Adelaide or the Flinders University of South Australia to benefit.*
>
> *Both Universities, and the Medical Faculty of each, have been advised of the terms of the Trust and we did seek from them any submissions they wished to make in support of their organization's selection by the Estate Trustees. A photocopy of the responses from both bodies is enclosed for your perusal.*
>
> *The response of the University of Adelaide is surprisingly brief.*

In paragraph two the condition relating to use of the funds for the expansion of the 'art' of teaching is referred to and in particular the shortcomings of the existing situation are acknowledged.

In this regard, the University of Adelaide appear to be relating the 'teaching art' to the existing staff and not to the student population as required by the words used in Clause 6 of the Will 'as in particular the training and education of graduates to qualify them in the principles and practice of teaching'.

It would however be only reasonable to note that any action to redress the situation described by Dr Heaslip in his Will as 'Lecturers who had been given no training as teachers' must commence at some point. This could very well be that initially funds are utilized to upgrade the abilities of existing lecturing staff in this regard.

Paragraph 3 refers to curriculum reviews conducted in 1969 and 1983. A copy of the 1983 review has been included. In relation to this, it is clearly stated that it is the School's intention to produce an undifferentiated graduate. This aspect particularly accords with Dr Heaslip's views expressed in Clause 7 (d).

The curative aspect of medicine is referred to in Paragraph 1 (e) of the report.

It is noted that, at the end of Paragraph 3 the University of Adelaide states 'the aims and objectives of the Medical Curriculum of the University of Adelaide are consistent with the principles expressed by Mr Heaslip in Clause 7 of his Will'.

The response of Flinders University of South Australia is far more extensive and a copy of this, together with the appendices referred to therein are also enclosed.

Flinders' submission claims in Paragraphs 1 and 2 that, because of the manner in which the Medical School was created, they had certain advantages over other Schools created on the historical basis of grafting them onto existing teaching hospitals. This would appear to be accord with the wording in Clause 6 'as efficient as possible'.

Paragraph 2.1 refers to the creation of the current curriculum by persons interested in educational reform. In particular, the basic philosophy expressed in Paragraphs 2.2 (f) would appear to be in direct accord with the views expressed in Clause 7 (c) and (d).

Part 4 of the submission specifically deals with the question of medical education and the improvement of teaching capabilities of the staff. It is this aspect that is at the heart of the Trust objectives. The inference contained in Paragraph 4.3, that the Trust could fund the re-instatement of the post of Lecturer in Medical Education is in direct opposition to the words in the Will 'nor for the establishment of permanent facilities such as Professorial Chairs, Departments or Units'. This inference, if correct, need not be of any great concern as the Trust Fund Trustees are charged with the responsibility to oversee the correct expenditure of the funds and can naturally overcome this type of use.

However, the more important aspect of this is that the Flinders University has in the past seen the need, so evident to the late Dr Heaslip and have endeavoured to overcome the shortcoming and wish to do so in the future.

In view of the above and the material supplied by both of the Universities, it would appear that the Flinders University may be the one that should be considered by the Trustees to benefit, and they appear to be more in accord with the late Dr Heaslip's wishes than Adelaide.

This conclusion of course, is to some extent coloured by the fact that the Flinders University did supply far more detail than did Adelaide.

The W.G. Heaslip Estate Trustees adopted the recommendation that the Heaslip Bequest be transferred to Flinders University, and they appointed Trust Fund Trustees to be responsible for disbursing funds in accordance with the provisions stipulated in the will.

Flinders University submission to executors

When Flinders University was notified by the executors of the opportunity to submit a proposal for the bequest outlined in the will of W.G. Heaslip, the medical school had recently been visited by the General Medical Council (GMC) of the United Kingdom. The GMC conducted a formal accreditation of the Flinders Medical course to ensure that the providers of the course, its curriculum and teaching methodology, were consistent with the standards required for graduates to be registered as medical practitioners in the UK. Prior to this visit, the Flinders Medical Program had received interim accreditation with the GMC on condition that the course would conform to GMC standards.

Until the Australian Medical Council was established in 1985, graduates of Australian medical schools were required to become Registered Medical Practitioners with the State Medical Board where they were conducting practice.

The Flinders Medical Program was approved by the GMC and Flinders Medical graduates became registered throughout Australia and overseas. The GMC submission was the source document for the Flinders University submission to the trustees of Gordon's estate. The key factors highlighted by Flinders included:

- Teaching support and training for clinical academics.
- Integration of teaching and research with clinical care.
- Emphasis on preventive medicine and general practice.

Flinders' ability to provide integrated teaching and clinical services was a result of the State Government's decision to establish Flinders University and a co-located teaching hospital and medical school in 1965 – Flinders Medical Centre (FMC) (Bright Committee of Enquiry into the Delivery of health Services in SA, 1970–73). This led to the establishment of the South Australian Health Commission and regionalising of health services.

FMC incorporated teaching and research facilities in a building complex that included a tertiary hospital with comprehensive diagnostic and treatment facilities. FMC was an integrated academic and health service centre for the southern region of Adelaide. University-appointed professors and academic staff were responsible for clinical services alongside teaching and research in the complete range of health needs. This included primary care and preventive medicine.

W.G. Heaslip wrote, 'The existing separation between research workers and clinicians must be removed so that there may be a maximum use of clinical data, maximum applications of clinical research findings, and a more intelligent and orderly direction of research' (*Medical Journal of Australia*, 6 July 1946). This was the ethos underpinning the integration of the Flinders Medical School with FMC.

Implementation of the Heaslip Bequest at Flinders University

When the Heaslip bequest was received in 1985, the Flinders Medical Program had been operating for over a decade. The bequest funds were transferred to a Heaslip trust fund within Flinders University, with trustees appointed to ensure that funds were allocated in accordance with the wishes and conditions outlined by Gordon.

Provisos for expenditure of the Heaslip Bequest by Flinders University were that funds should be directed to projects to improve efficiency of clinical teaching with particular emphasis on preventive medicine and general practice.

Initial projects funded by the Heaslip Trust fund were the study of the teaching of surgery, provision of Heaslip Fellowships for medical graduates to improve the efficiency of teaching in general practice, and curriculum development of study programs in preventative health directed toward improving health outcomes.

Teaching surgery

Surgical teaching encompasses not just learning procedural techniques, but also an understanding of the disease processes that lead to surgical interventions and how they might be prevented.

Traditionally, surgical teaching was conducted in teaching hospitals where patients were available for examination by students, and procedures like suturing and fracture management could be taught alongside lectures and tutorials about disease processes.

In modern hospitals like FMC, patients are rarely available for bedside teaching because their length of hospital stay is short, they are often confined to specialised units like ICU, and due consideration for patient privacy and comfort limits the extent to which they can be available for teaching students.

The first project undertaken under the Heaslip Bequest was an investigation into the teaching of surgery, conducted by the first Heaslip Fellow Dr David Prideaux. The investigation clarified the way core surgical knowledge, skills and understanding could be integrated into each year of the curriculum together with assessment processes that validated student competency.

The engagement of practising surgeons in this teaching process was crucial and arose from case-study methodologies that required surgeons to coordinate relevant experts in pre-clinical sciences, pathology, and primary care in tutorials that considered the overall management of a patient whose case notes were available [with permission] for teaching purposes.

An important innovation that was introduced into the curriculum by Professor Jim Toouli, a surgeon at Flinders, was a way of assessing clinical skills through a process of Objective Structured Clinical Examination (OSCE). The OSCE involves a dozen or so 'patients' at specific stations in a large room; students are asked at each station to assess the patient visually and undertake a clinical test or task. Students have five minutes to complete the task, record an answer, and move on to the next station.

The OSCE has proven to be a reliable and standardised process of validating clinical skills. This assessment process is now applied in a range of clinical disciplines in the health sciences around Australia.

The combination of case studies and OSCE examination proved to be an effective approach for teaching students about all aspects of surgery, and importantly engaged surgeons as mentors in curriculum design and execution.

Heaslip Fellows and general practice

Teaching and training students in primary care (general practice) is a challenge for medical schools. From inception, the Flinders Medical Program involved GPs who supervised students attending patient consultations in the GPs' consulting rooms. The GP discussed the role of primary care in overall health management and was important in guiding career choices as students progressed through the medical course.

Many GPs were enthusiastic about teaching, and they sought assistance in refining their teaching skills and appraising student capability. Accordingly, a program of Heaslip Fellowships was created. Heaslip Fellows were medical graduates who received a grant to support them in studying teaching in general practice and ways of improving the quality and effectiveness of teaching. There has been a succession of Heaslip Fellows studying specific aspects of teaching with emphasis on general practice and curriculum development consistent with the stipulations in the Heaslip Bequest.

Future directions for the Heaslip Bequest

During the 40 years of support from the Heaslip Bequest, the Flinders Medical Program has evolved to embrace medical training in rural and remote locations and has modified the course structure accordingly. The impact of the bequest has been to improve teaching efficiency in surgery, support general practice development, and contribute to assessment of clinical skills.

Gordon Heaslip believed that medical education was the key to changing the health system so that doctors would practise preventive medicine alongside disease management. Clause 8 of the Heaslip Bequest states:

> THE TRUST FUND TRUSTEES WILL BEAR IN MIND [that] THE MEDICAL UNDERGRADUATE SHOULD HAVE EMPHASIS ON PREVENTIVE MEDICINE [rather than curative] AND WILL BEAR THIS IN MIND AND

EMPHASISE IT WHENEVER ANY OPPORTUNITY TO DO SO PRESENTS ITSELF.

It is a sentiment echoed by the medical deans of Australia and New Zealand:

> *Whilst access to acute care when needed is vital, we need to focus far more on preventative, early and on-going care for chronic conditions, which is provided in community-based settings close to, and sometimes in, the patient's home.*
>
> *We need more doctors in primary care. All doctors need to: practice preventative healthcare, understand the impact of the social determinants of health on chronic and co-morbid conditions, and support their patients in taking a greater role in self-care both physically and mentally. (From 'Training Tomorrow's Doctors: all pulling in the right direction', September 2021, p. 5.)*

With assistance from the Heaslip Bequest, the Flinders Medical School delivered improvements in health outcomes by way of integrated teaching, research, and patient care. Preventive medicine was delivered through large-scale trials in hypertension management (Chalmers, Wing), reduction in post-operative sepsis in gastrointestinal surgery (Watts, McDonald), reductions in pre-term births (McDonald, O'Loughlin), and improved sight by way of cataract surgery (Coster).

Historically, preventive medicine was referred to as medical hygiene. In recent times the terms 'preventive' and 'preventative' have been used interchangeably to denote medical care that prevents progression to disease. This includes public health and social factors in disease prevention.

Impact of the bequest on Flinders Medical curriculum

When Flinders University first received the Heaslip Bequest in 1985, the full complement of teaching staff had been recruited, the curriculum was running smoothly, graduates were entering medical practice, and some were pursuing higher degrees in Australia and overseas.

Flinders Medical Centre was the crucible for integrating teaching, research and patient care that attracted a faculty of medical academics from Australia and overseas to lead the Flinders Medical School. This Flinders academic medical faculty was able to fulfil the aspirations of Gordon Heaslip to improve clinical teaching efficiency and emphasise preventive medicine in terms of treatments that prevented progression of disease and maintained health.

However, from the 1980s, Federal Government intrusion into medical education became an ongoing issue for all medical schools. At Flinders, specific factors threatened the viability of the medical program:

- In 1985, a 10 per cent reduction in admissions to medical schools was imposed by the Commonwealth Government. In response, Flinders established a clinical school in the Northern Territory and commenced its rural medical training program in South Australia.
- Funding arrangements for teaching hospitals, general practice, and higher education were rearranged around the implementation of Medicare and the Dawkins Funding for Tertiary Education. These 'reforms' resulted in formation of the South Australian Department of Health in lieu of the SA Health Commission, and new funding arrangements for SA public hospitals, universities and medical schools, fracturing the integration of teaching, research and patient care at FMC.

This occurred around the departure of foundation professors and heads of department from the mid-1990s. Some retired, others moved to prestige positions interstate; a few continued to sustain the ethos of FMC by their leadership in South Australian and national health programs.

- Quotas for medical admissions under the Dawkins reforms reverted from a state-based quota to a national competitive selection process. These reductions were a strategy for reducing demand on medical services in a belief that medical practitioners were partly responsible for the increasing costs of the health budget.

The restrictions were eased in 2000 when new medical schools opened.

How many medical graduates are required?
At the end of 2020, 3656 students graduated from Australian medical schools; 83.9 per cent were domestic graduates and 52 per cent were female. Based on enrolments it is estimated that 3910 students will graduate in 2024, taking account of an attrition rate of 2.9 per cent since enrolment.

In 2020 there were 104,000 medical doctors and specialists in Australia; these comprised 31,000 GPs and 36,000 specialists. Of these 104,000 practitioners:

- More than 80,000 worked in major cities, 20,000 in regions and 1500 in remote areas.
- 46,000 worked in hospitals and 35,000 in private practices.
- About 70 per cent gained their qualifications in Australia and 45 per cent were born in Australia. (Based on Medical Deans of Australia and New Zealand Student Statistics Report 2021 and www.health.gov.au/topics/doctors-and-specialists)

Notwithstanding changes in enrolment patterns, the numbers of practitioners in Australia will increase only slightly over the next few years. In 2023 there were insufficient numbers of general practitioners to satisfy existing demands generally, and particularly in regional and remote Australia.

We are in the midst of a health crisis in Australia, mainly because of the excessive demand for emergency admissions to hospitals. These are a consequence of improvements in medical treatments, health maintenance programs and public health.

The solution to this crisis is a reform in primary care, which will prevent the need for hospital admissions. Thus, medical and health education should be planning to produce graduates who will contribute to the reforms in primary care that are underway with government support to provide for future national health needs.

Australia's Future Health Policies envisage a primary care team comprising general practitioners, medical specialists, nursing and allied health jointly delivering coordinated care for all patients and members of the community. This has many implications for medical and health training and education.

Life expectancy

Life expectancy is a demographic that expresses the average number of years a person of a given sex and age could be expected to live throughout life, assuming age-specific death rates experienced throughout their life.

In 1900, the average life expectancy was about 45 years. In 1950 it was 66.5 years; by 2010 it had increased to 81.83 years.

Factors that have extended life have changed over the decades

Between 1900 and postwar in 1950, increased life expectancy was the result of improvements in maternal and child health, vaccination, anti-biotics, health hygiene (waste, food quality), and health promotion (anti-smoking campaigns, better diets).

From 1950, the dominant causes of mortality were cardiovascular disease, cancer, diabetes chronic respiratory disease, inherited and mental health conditions.

Improvements in mortality between 1960 and 2010 have been associated with improvements in determinants of health (socio-economic status, education, productivity), but improved treatments for premature mortality have been the major contributor to increased life expectancy.

Cardiovascular diseases [myocardial infarct and stroke] were the dominant causes of premature mortality immediately after WW II. These continued to rise until the results of research clearly indicated that smoking, high blood pressure, obesity, diabetes and high cholesterol were major contributing causes to premature mortality. Initiatives to combat premature cardiovascular mortality commenced from 1960 and included:

- Establishing coronary care units to treat acute myocardial infarcts and develop coronary artery bypass surgery to improve blood supply to heart muscle.
- Treating hypertension with effective agents that reduced blood pressure to 'normal' levels.
- Reducing excess cholesterol with 'statin' drugs that impair cholesterol metabolism.

These initiatives were associated with a reduction of mortality between 1970 when cardiovascular diseases were responsible for 55 per cent of all deaths until 2015 when cardiovascular mortality reduced to 29 per cent.

In this period, treatments with medications in primary care and the availability of joint replacements, cataract surgery and improvements in lifestyle have increased mobility and quality of life.

By 2020, it was apparent that the causes of mortality had evolved.

While cardiovascular disease remains the most prominent underlying cause of mortality of males in 2023/4, dementia has emerged as the most prominent underlying cause of death in women. In men, dementia is second to cardiovascular disease as underlying cause of death.

Thus, successful treatment of the common underlying risk factors of mortality means that medical treatment has prolonged life expectancy to the situation where underlying causes of ageing, i.e. senescence of tissues in various body organs, is now emerging as the major cause of disability and mortality from dementia.

Preventive health, disease prevention, disease management, public health, and social determinants of health

All the above factors have combined to bring about a life expectancy in 2024 that has progressed to the point where continued access to medications to prevent disease progression is required to maintain current life expectancy.

Primary care, incorporating general practice, is the element of the health system that is best able to coordinate and deliver improved population health outcomes.

Hospital care is necessary for treating serious illness and for undertaking procedures that maintain health and mobility. The standards of modern treatments in hospital most frequently result in successful outcomes and patients are discharged to resume living in the community. Sometimes hospitalisation is the first manifestation of an ongoing health condition.

Australia's health system is under stress in large part because of the rates of hospital admissions of people living with ongoing conditions like angina, heart failure, diabetes, asthma and many other eminently 'manageable' conditions. These people are not seeking or receiving timely medical care to prevent their condition deteriorating and, as a result, progressing to emergency hospital admission.

Role of medical schools in the Australian health system
Medical schools are responsible for producing doctors to work within the health system. Traditionally, clinical training is focused on teaching hospitals and periods of secondment to general practices affiliated with medical schools. This clinical apprenticeship occurs within the Medicare system of health care. Since medical schools are training future doctors, they need to be aware that Australia's health system is in crisis and should be pursuing strategies in primary care that can achieve improved population health outcomes, while reducing emergency admissions to hospitals.

The solution to the health crisis revolves around supporting people and the community to maintain a sense of wellbeing while participating in community activities (*A Community-Powered NHS, Future focused primary health care: Australia's Primary Care 10-year Plan 2022–2032*).

Flinders Medical Centre participated in the implementation of research into patient care. Much of this research was directed at improving treatments for common diseases, especially cardiovascular, respiratory, infectious diseases, and making surgery safer. In addition, Flinders was involved in community public health programs like safer cities and general practice. When FMC was commissioned, it was equipped with the latest laboratory and imaging technology, which improved diagnostic capability and enabled angiography, keyhole surgery, cataract lens replacements, and prosthetic joint replacements.

Disease treatments evolve to disease prevention

Cardiovascular disease and hypertension were major foci of research for FMC academics between 1975 and 2008. Treatments for hypertension became available from the 1950s but it was not until the 1970s that population studies clearly demonstrated that treating people with elevated blood pressure significantly reduced deaths from cardiovascular disease. FMC cardiology played a leading role in conducting research into the most effective dosing regimens from among the many pharmaceutical products that became available for treatment of hypertension. Importantly, they identified the optimal levels of systolic and diastolic blood pressure that warranted treatment.

These investigations were prospective studies that enrolled people with hypertension and followed them for many years to confirm the most effective regimens that reduced heart attacks and strokes.

The treatment of hypertension and availability of interventions to prevent cardiovascular disease has created an older population who are living comfortably with their chronic condition. A similar pathway to a chronic condition occurs with diabetes, lung disease (asthma, bronchitis), degenerative bone disease, sun exposure diseases, and many other conditions that have become dependent on modern health care to prevent premature mortality.

In summary, the common causes of death arise from conditions that are manifest in early life as illnesses or risk factors. These can be managed with medications or lifestyle changes to prevent complications. When complications occur, preventive treatments in primary care can avert serious disease requiring emergency hospitalisation. Sometimes, serious diseases require hospitalisation, but patients usually return to their community life, albeit with ongoing review and medication to prevent further deterioration.

Judicious management of people with risk factors and a chronic health problem has been shown by Flinders in National Coordinated Care trials (1994–2004) to diminish emergency hospital admissions, improve quality of life, and reduce the burden of hospital admissions. Government policies and funding in primary care and strengthening Medicare have created the opportunity for Flinders to provide further leadership to achieve population health outcomes consistent with in health care, based on existing strengths in Flinders University and relationships with governments and health providers.

Opportunity for Flinders to contribute to health outcomes and preventive health consistent with Heaslip aspirations
Flinders has contributed to increasing life expectancy through research and implementation of strategies for people with risk factors to be supported through life with treatments that prevent premature death and disability. The challenge for the future is to evolve primary health care into a system that is focused on health maintenance, preventive health measures, and patient satisfaction in their contribution to a productive society.

At the time of writing, few medical schools around Australia appear to be taking leadership positions in health reform. Research in general practice is being conducted with practice development grants by groups of practices supported by the College of General Practice and the AMA.

Specific initiatives

The shape of future health care is evident from policies outlined in 'Future focused primary health care: Australia's Primary Health Care 10 Year Plan 2022–2032', Commonwealth of Australia (Department of Health) 2022.

The foundations for health reform include:

- Voluntary patient registration encouraging an ongoing relationship between patients and their general practice. The practice will be committed to supporting the enrolled patient through a care plan that includes access to allied health and pharmaceutical services.
- Inclusion of allied health in providing a range of services on the care plan that will be funded and available in regional and remote locations. This will include funded MBS items for allied health professionals' participation in multidisciplinary case conferences.
- MBS-funded telehealth, which allows for telephone and video consultations.

These policies provide the opportunity for Flinders to devise ways of integrating health disciplines into a framework that delivers improved health outcomes for patients and the community.

During 2024, the Australian Government has implemented policies for strengthening Medicare that include expanded Medicare funding for long telephone consultations, additional nursing and allied health consultations for people with chronic and complex conditions, and general practice and aged care incentives that fund regular health assessments, care plans and visits for residential aged care homes.

There are clearly insufficient general practitioners to satisfy the demand in primary care for consultations that will prevent emergency admissions to hospital and implement effective preventive health care. Central to the success of these reforms is the incorporation of nursing and allied health alongside general practitioners into the process of care planning and support of people with chronic health issues.

In October 2024 the Australian Government's Department of Health and Aged Care released the final report of a Scope of Practice Review 'Unleashing the Potential of Our Health Workforce' that provides a pathway for multidisciplinary teams to be supported by legislation, funding and recognition of the skills of the full range of health professionals.

These policies provide the opportunity for Flinders to devise ways of integrating health disciplines into a framework that delivers improved health outcomes for patients and the community, fulfilling Gordon Heaslip's aspirations of implementing preventive health in the community and reinforcing primary health care.

It is recommended that the trustees of the Flinders University Heaslip Bequest fund allocate funds for the coordination of medical, nursing and allied health teaching and research programmes to achieve national health reforms.

NATIONAL HEALTH.

By W. G. Heaslip,
Adelaide.

And if we speak our minds, it is because the fascist threat to civilization, with its lies and its propaganda and its blasphemous hatred of objectivity, makes any suppression of the truth or suggestion of the false of which we might be guilty a betrayal of ultimate standards which are everywhere in peril.

Victor Gollancz.

It is evident from the Federal Government's proposal to nationalize the medical service that some of our politicians are at last aware of the importance of the national health. They apparently believe that the standard could and should be improved. There is no doubt that they are right. The untimely dead sent to their graves by preventible accident or disease, the inmates of hospitals and institutions who suffer needlessly through ignorance and poverty, and the deformed and disabled, so many of whom are living memorials to ineptitude, all bear witness to the imperfection of our national health and to the inadequacy of our health services.

Let it be stated at once that the medical profession cannot of itself supply what is required to produce optimal health. Nor will nationalizing the medical service alone produce the desired result. The war has shown, particularly in England, that the public health may improve dramatically when the number of medical practitioners has been drastically reduced and the remainder are working under great difficulties. This improvement was due mainly to three factors, which were: (a) movement of slum-dwellers to rural areas, (b) more equitable distribution of and improvement in nature of diet, and (c) elimination of unemployment amongst poor and rich and young and old. None of these is primarily a medical matter. But it appears that such diverse problems as employment of the idle, slum clearance, nutritionally balanced diets, unemployment, decentralization, and elimination of poverty all have a direct bearing on national health. The subject is as complex as the matter of improvement is urgent, and real success will be achieved only by a concerted effort of the whole community.

The articles and letters, which have appeared in medical journals and in the lay Press since the proposal to nationalize medical services was made, demonstrate that neither the public nor the profession fully appreciates the problems involved in improving the national health. This article is an attempt to state and examine briefly some of the basic aspects of the subject, with the detached interest of the spectator who has been a player. If certain statements are found to be provocative, they are not made maliciously, but only to emphasize certain facts which appear to have been neglected previously.

The Medical Profession.

There should be no need to state that the profession should exist for the sole purpose of improving and maintaining the health of the people. Nevertheless it is necessary to remind both the public and the profession that this is the case. While it is well that members should remember that their profession originated from witchcraft and superstition, it is high time they realized that they are public servants and not high priests.

Unfortunately the profession is not at present solely concerned with the people's health. Only a few of the members realize that they are public servants. Possibly still less are intelligently active in trying to improve matters. The provision of an adequate curative service, with some attempts at prevention, is not enough. What is required is that an adequate curative service be made available to everyone, irrespective of his position geographically, financially or morally, and that prevention be implemented to the limit of available knowledge.

It is comforting to remember the great advances that have been made in medicine and surgery in the past century. It is, however, distinctly unpleasant to realize that the public is becoming aware of the shortcomings of the profession, and that the politicians have taken the lead in initiating reforms. The war has blasted open the windows of the mind for many people. The winds of enlightenment have been sweeping in for some years. The "mysteries" of health are doomed along with the "mysteries" of finance. People are becoming increasingly aware that the fundamental right of man is his right to an adequate share of what this world has produced, including man's knowledge and skill in preventing disease and disability.

It is becoming obvious that health is much more dependent on social structure than on medical practice, and that education is more important than medication. It is now common knowledge that disease and disability are mainly due to ignorance and poverty. It cannot be very long before the profession will be asked why it remains satisfied with attempting to cure disease which it should have prevented. It may well be accused openly, as it is now tacitly by the reformers, of failing, *inter alia*: (a) to demand a form of society which would permit everyone to have the chance of maximum health; (b) to demand a system and standard of education which would fulfil the requirements of optimum health; and (c) to educate and train its members adequately.

Appendix

No honest, educated member of the profession would deny these failures, which are the outcome of its basic failure to realize and to take its proper place in society. This place of high standing is attained only in the office of defender of the people's health. If the profession is to reach this goal the members will have to indulge in considerable realism, honesty, and self-education. When they have done this, the following may happen.

(i) They may realize that they are entitled to no special rights or privileges other than those essential for the maintenance of an adequate service available to everyone.

(ii) They may accept the fact that it is their responsibility to prevent every avoidable illness, accident or disability and to alleviate or cure what cannot be prevented.

(iii) They may proudly acknowledge that they are public servants, and cease to be pediars of dubious cures.

(iv) They may appreciate fully that their fellow men rely on them for leadership in all matters pertaining to health.

These fruits of realism, honesty and idealism form the background to all future planning, and the basis of any successful proposal for improving the medical service and raising the status of the profession. It is painfully evident at present that the profession has failed to take the lead and that it has lost touch with reality. It has forgotten or ignored the fundamental reason for its existence. This is well illustrated by what members have written in discussing the proposed reforms. It can be said of most of those supporting, as well as all of those opposing, a nationalized service that they are more concerned with the effects on members of the profession than the effects on the national health.

The Public.

Acting on behalf of the public, the Minister for Health is advised by a Parliamentary Joint Committee. The advice and recommendations it tenders are therefore not coloured by party politics. The members of the committee are very well informed on the varying aspects of public health. Unfortunately they are not so well informed on matters of medical practice. To remedy this defect the Minister should also have an advisory committee composed mainly of doctors in active practice. At present the political reformers, as part of the public they represent, share with it the disabilities due to lack of knowledge and expert advice. The recent free medicine bill was an example of this.

For a great many years the sick in mind, as well as the sick in body, have been given infusions instead of instruction, and pills instead of propaganda. The result is a demand for medicine out of a bottle to cure both their ills and their ignorance. We can agree with the principle of not making the individual pay for his medicine, since we have largely ceased to regard illness as a form of divine retribution. But any honest doctor would have advised the Minister for Health that only a small number of drugs are curative; that nearly all the mixtures which are taken have only a psychological effect; and that, while the people want medicine, it is not medicine, in most cases, that they need. If the bill were intended to lessen the taking of preparations not prescribed by a doctor, the honest medical adviser would have pointed out that this pernicious practice is due mainly to ignorance, partly to the expense of getting a prescription, and partly to the infamous propaganda from the vendors of patent medicines. It is to the credit of the profession that it has protested against the traffic in patent medicines, but so far no government has had the courage to prevent it. The public, as a consequence, has become sickness-conscious instead of being health-conscious.

Therefore, while it is desirable that the public should discard its ancient attitude of awe-struck veneration and should learn to regard the members of the profession as responsible for ensuring an adequate medical service, it is essential for the public representatives in Parliament to remember that the profession alone can provide expert advice in matters of medical practice. It should need no further demonstration that the public is not in a position to choose wisely either its medicine or its doctor. Since it is not even in a position to know what it needs, it rightly expects its expert representatives to supply a health service which is wholly adequate and available.

The public ignorance in itself constitutes a demand for reform without delay. Since manpower is the basic wealth of the nation, there is an economic as well as a humanitarian reason for haste. Moreover, consideration of what is involved, in the provision of an adequate health service for everyone, will show that, no matter how great an effort we make, the task will be lengthy as well as arduous. It will need the combined efforts of public, politicians and profession if there is to be success. The people will have to learn and to pay, the doctors will have to work and to lead, while the politicians will have to become statesmen and provide the necessary reforms.

The Problem of Adequacy.

The chief difficulties of making the service adequate can be briefly outlined under the headings of prevention, medical competence, material facilities, and organisation.

Prevention.

From every point of view prevention is better than cure. Therefore the keystone of an adequate service must be prevention. The first step is to ensure that each individual has a sound mind and a healthy body. To achieve this, the body must be given suitable housing, food, clothing, sanitation, employment, recreation and medical attention from birth to death. These are merely basic requirements. For the mind there must be also a suitable education. Such an education would involve practical and theoretical instruction on how to keep healthy, to work, to think, to play, to govern one's actions on a rational basis, and to recognize, control and usefully express emotional impulses.

Making these basic requirements available involves both give and take. It would not be sufficient that the means of education be provided. The instruction must be given by proficient teachers, and must be received by each individual in suitable circumstances and under hygienic conditions. Likewise the essentials for a healthy body must not only be supplied. There must also be the opportunity for everyone to take and use them. They must be available to those in isolated places as well as to those in the city, and to the poor as well as to the rich.

There must also be an active, continuous campaign of public education (propaganda), dealing with both active and passive prevention. People must be made health-conscious. At present the fear of disease, which arises from ignorance and pernicious propaganda, is probably as great an evil as any disease entity in Australia. At the same time much existing disease and disability is the direct result of ignorance. The provision of education is a matter for the politicians, but the profession has the responsibility of ensuring that the public gets the right education.

The profession must also make prevention the keynote of members' training. Most of the disabilities that can be cured can be prevented. Every medical student should be taught that: (a) each disability should be investigated from the aspect of prevention as well as correction; (b) every endeavour and resource should be used to discover the causes of an illness or accident; (c) not only the primary, but also the contributing causes, should be discovered and removed.

Finally, to secure maximum prevention, it will be necessary for the profession and the politicians to devise a form of service which will make it possible to have the following desiderata:

1. The cooperation of the dental, veterinary, physiotherapy and other professions, and of the auxiliary services, such as entomology and optometry.

2. The utilization of adequately trained health officers, engineers, architects and others to deal with such matters as town-planning, water supplies, sanitation, size and situation of factories, hospitals, schools and sanatoria, and food-planning.

3. Facilities of all types to enable (a) necessary preventive research to be done; (b) every individual to be dentally and medically examined at regular, frequent

intervals; (c) every expectant mother to be made competent in the care, management, and feeding of mother, fœtus, baby and child; (d) every woman, who so desires, to become a mother without shame or degradation; and (e) every doctor to implement such measures as may be required to prevent ill health and physical or mental disability.

These few notes will suffice to show that implementing prevention to the limit of available knowledge will provide a firm basis for a sound national health service.

Medical Competence.

Apart from neglect of preventive measures, it is regrettably plain that the standard of competence reached and maintained by the profession as a whole is not as high as it might be. Nor can it reach the desired height until the whole medical service, including the teaching and training of members, is reorganized. Every member must be taught and trained from the beginning to the end of his career. He must be made and kept as competent as possible. A practicable scheme of training in a reorganized service is outlined below.

There will have to be sufficient doctors to allow each one to attend post-graduate lectures and demonstrations at regular intervals, and also to allow time for study and reading, for investigation of significant phenomena, to record interesting or important data, and to prepare articles and reports.

The existing separation between research workers and clinicians must be removed so that there may be maximum use of clinical data, maximum application of research findings, and a more intelligent and orderly direction of research.

Medical competence is dependent on others besides the members of the profession. In particular the standard of nursing practice must be raised to and maintained at the highest possible level. Nursing services must be extended and improved. In addition there is the whole lay staff associated with medical services. Dressers, cleaners, cooks, technicians, dietitians and others must all be trained and provided for, so that they are able at all times to give the highest possible standard of service. Until medical competence reaches the highest attainable standard, our health services cannot be adequate.

Material Facilities.

No service can be adequate unless it is provided with the best facilities. At present our health facilities are far from being the best. Our hospital accommodation is short of our needs and our hospitals range from good to bad. Design, size, situation and equipment must all be studied continuously and, whenever necessary, modernization must be effected. Siting and grouping of hospitals is at present mainly bad. Nearly all modern, well-equipped ones are found in the heart of a large town or city, instead of in an area away from smoke, dust, noise, crowds and other buildings. All that is required in the cities is a sufficient number of emergency and casualty stations to deal with patients needing immediate help.

Facilities for associated services must be extended and modernized. Country centres should be supplied with buildings and equipment for dental, physiotherapy, radiology and pathology units. Research facilities must be brought up to date and extended. Mobile research units should be provided so that any epidemic, in any place, can be promptly and efficiently investigated *in situ*.

Clinics, convalescent depots and sanatoria must be supplied where required. It may be noted, however, that the necessity for such units would decrease rapidly with the increased practice of prevention. For example, the elimination of poverty and its contingent evils would make it comparatively easy to control, and practically to eliminate, such diseases as syphilis, tuberculosis and rheumatic fever. It is only because of ignorance and apathy that diphtheria is not already controlled.

This may seem an expensive programme, but any expense directed to preventing disease is a good national investment.

Organization.

Under the heading of "Prevention" a few matters involving organization are listed. These and others mentioned elsewhere make it clear that an adequate health service will need most careful organization. There must be sufficient elasticity to meet any advance in knowledge or any other emergency, and to deal effectively with it. No cumbrous, unwieldy, administrative machine, which is incapable of acting swiftly or of accepting responsibility, will serve. There must be a complete absence of any sort of dictatorship from either above or below.

It is quite obvious that the government must have the full cooperation of doctors, dentists, and a large number of other experts. It is equally obvious that if those employed in the service are to give the necessary time and attention to their work, and to their own physical and mental fitness, they must be paid a sufficient salary. To ensure equitable staffing and facilities for all localities, hospitals *et cetera*, a Commonwealth controlling body will be necessary. Since there must be coordination of non-medical with primarily medical projects, a central coordinating body will be needed. On the other hand, local administration, with full authority and responsibility, is essential to maximum efficiency in any department, locality or unit.

Executive officers should be specially trained in health matters. In no circumstances should a medical officer hold a purely administrative post. All such posts should be filled by election and should not carry a salary in excess of that paid to medical officers. Every other means should be used to avoid the creation of a single unnecessary administrative post, so that there may be the utmost simplicity of organization. This will produce greater efficiency and will combat the tendency of the administration to grow complex and, at certain points, remote.

No attempt is made here to outline a sample organization, as there are many possible ways of introducing the service. It may be started in certain areas and later extended to others. Social reforms may be started prior to nationalization of medical services, and so on. However, the type of organization which is required is essentially cooperative, as indicated below.

The Problem of Availability.

In passing it should be noted that a separate set of problems exists in the making of health services available to the native populations of attached or mandated territories. A survey of the remainder of our own aborigines will show that it may be stated, as a guiding principle, that no government is entitled to take over the management of any native community, unless it is prepared and determined to provide adequate educational and health services forthwith.

Within Australia the chief factor affecting availability is the economic one. At present the services of doctors, given free to non-paying patients, are paid for by an overcharge on the rich. Even so there is always a section of the poorer classes who cannot obtain service, free or otherwise. For example, the "free" service at hospital out-patient departments can be quite expensive for the patient who has to forfeit a half or whole day's pay to get it. Then there are the employees to whom the venereal disease clinic is not available because it is not open when the patient is free to attend. Application for time off in these cases would probably mean loss of employment. There is also the wage-earner to whom hospital facilities are not available because of helpless dependants, and the mother with a family of young children whom she cannot leave because there is no one to look after them. In these cases even pregnancy and confinement can be an acute embarrassment. This situation is commonly found amongst the middle classes in the economic scale also, and is a definite factor in retarding our needed increase of population. All too frequently desirable pathological or radiological investigations are not available because they are too expensive. It is clear that a service may be provided without its being available to everyone.

The lack of hospital accommodation, which is a disgrace to each of the governments concerned, becomes greater year by year. Even if sick people could be properly nursed at home it would not be fair to ask a woman to be confined in her home. In any case there are not sufficient doctors and nurses to give proper attention to patients confined to bed at home, and the shortage of nurses is now an acute problem. Moreover, there is a shortage of lay staff, at hospitals and institutions, which is also only partly due to war conditions. Poor pay and poor conditions are the main causes of all these shortages. They are also responsible for poor quality service. Any sort of cheeseparing economy in a health service is false economy and is incompatible with the availability of the service to everyone.

Another aspect of the problem in Australia is a small population scattered over a huge area. But with the perfecting of wireless communication and of air travel there is no longer any valid reason for service not being available, even in the most isolated spots.

From what has been written here and in the previous section, it is clear that to make an adequate service available to everyone means much more than nationalization of the medical service. It means reforming our educational system and, indeed, our whole social system. But the magnitude and complexity of the task do not mean that it is impossible or even impracticable. Given an early lead by the profession, the full backing of all our politicians, and the cooperation of the auxiliary services, there is no doubt that the public would fully support its leaders and within a generation would have a health service which would produce optimum national health.

A Practicable Service.

The following brief outline suggests a service which would prove practicable and would fulfil the objectives set out above.

Country Areas.

In the remoter parts there would be a series of strategically placed hospitals with one or two doctors, and at least one ambulance plane, available to each. Although small, these remote hospitals would be staffed and equipped for dealing with any probable emergency. Equipment would include effective transmitting and receiving sets.

Patients who could not be wholly treated at such remote hospitals would be evacuated to the nearest rural hospital. Each of the latter would be staffed by at least three doctors and a resident trainee. Where there were only three doctors one must have specialized in surgery and be a competent radiographer; another must have specialized as a physician and be a capable anæsthetist; while the third must have specialized in obstetrics and be able to do routine pathology investigations. With more doctors these specialty and auxiliary services would be more easily provided. This would ensure a fairly complete service for the area. Patients requiring lengthy or specialized treatment or investigation would be transferred to the appropriate base hospital.

Urban Areas.

In urban areas, instead of the flying doctor, would be the factory doctor attending to one or more industrial units, and the emergency doctors at the casualty hospitals. The counterpart of the rural hospital would be the suburban hospital, similarly staffed by a group of doctors selected to give as complete a service as possible to the area covered. The medical staffs of rural and suburban hospitals, together with the emergency, flying and factory doctors, would comprise the equivalent of the present general practitioners.

The casualty hospitals would serve the purpose of a clearing station and would be sited accordingly. They would be staffed and equipped to do all types of emergency work, including resuscitation, operation and treatment of shock, but would have only sufficient beds for those who could not be moved safely. Outside the cities there would be base hospitals for the treatment of chronic, infectious and other special diseases, and for the investigation of obscure conditions. Sanatoria and convalescent depots would not necessarily be in urban areas.

General.

Wherever there was need, dental, pre-natal, child welfare and other clinics, crèches, laboratories, radiological centres and similar services would be provided. Consultation rooms would normally be at the hospital. Where the latter was distant from the main body of people a consulting centre should be equipped at the most suitable site.

Treatment of patients at home should be reduced to a minimum. Out-patient departments would be practically abolished, since they are necessary only where proper hospital accommodation is not available and/or treatment is unsatisfactory. Where the latter is not merely a confession of failure by the doctor, the patient should be cared for in a hospital for chronic illness where he could work according to his ability.

Each doctor or group of doctors would be responsible for the health of the people in the area concerned.

Administration.

Flying doctors and the nearest rural hospital, emergency and factory doctors and the adjacent suburban hospital or hospitals, and base hospitals, singly or in groups, could each comprise a unit attending to its own internal affairs and conferring with other units as required. A committee representative of all sections of the unit should be the executive body. There would also be a coordinating committee for each State or similar area. It should consist of a representative of each of the various units and each of the various categories of staff. It would frame the general policy for the area from reports and estimates submitted by the constituent units.

The Commonwealth administrative staff should be as few as possible. There should be an advisory panel or committee representing all areas and aspects of the service, including building, engineering, supply, flying doctors and hospitals. An executive committee in conjunction with government representatives would frame the general policy. Each of the above representatives should be elected democratically. If possible there would be no "appointments".

Teaching and Training.

Teaching and training must be extended and modified to meet the requirements outlined above. The selection of teachers is of the utmost importance. It has never been realized, apparently, that the only people competent to judge the worth of a teacher are his students. At the end of each year every class should report on the suitability of its teacher. At present far too many student hours are wasted attending compulsory, useless lectures. No university lectures should be compulsory. If the teachers are satisfactory the students will attend.

There must be a revision of the curriculum. Botany and zoology could be replaced by a course of lectures and demonstrations in tropical medicine, given later in the course. The present course in physics should be replaced by a short course in biophysics. Anatomy and dissection should be started in first year. Some instruction in statistical methods should also be given in first year. The amount of time given to both biochemistry and *materia medica* could be reduced. The teaching of histology and pathology should be combined. The early study of physiology should be limited to its bearing on practical medicine, and that of pathology to the understanding and diagnosis of disease. Further study of these two subjects would be done later, as required. More time would be given to the study of prevention and psychiatry.

There is no need for the student to memorize the signs, symptoms and treatment of obscure or chronic conditions. They can be determined at one's convenience. Similarly, the treatment of most disabilities can await the establishment of diagnosis, and does not demand the memorizing of facts, charts, scales and figures. But more attention must be given to examination, observation and diagnosis, so as to prevent unnecessary hospitalization and loss of manpower. The treatment and diagnosis of emergencies must be known infallibly, as must the action and dosage of drugs used in or giving rise to emergencies.

A student should be accepted for training only on the recommendation of his previous teachers. With the application for admission to the service he should present a statement of his reasons for applying, and his conceptions of what medical service involves. On acceptance a salary sufficient for his needs would be paid to each student, and continuance of training would depend on progress and conduct. These matters would be decided by a committee composed of undergraduates and graduates.

At the end of two years (possibly less), completed satisfactorily, ward work would commence and would continue for at least three years, together with lectures and demonstrations. Set lectures would then cease, but the student would continue reading in certain fixed subjects and in others as desired for a further two years. The first of these would be spent as a resident officer at a base, suburban or rural hospital. The second would be spent as junior assistant attached to a rural or suburban hospital, or in three months of residence at a maternity, a casualty, an infectious diseases and a mental hospital. This would complete the first part of the course and the three degrees of Bachelor of Medicine, Bachelor of Surgery and Bachelor of Medical Science could be conferred on the deserving.

Study and training would continue for at least another three years as part of the course. Some of the trainees, in the first of these three years, would act as emergency, factory, and flying doctors; others would become senior assistants attached to rural or suburban hospitals. In the next two years all of the above group would transfer to base hospitals for completion of training in medicine or surgery. Those intending to specialize in obstetrics, infectious diseases, psychiatry, gynæcology et cetera would spend the three years attached to an appropriate hospital, for the first year at least as resident officers. Those who wished to become biochemists, or radiologists, or pathologists et cetera would commence work in the appropriate hospitals, laboratories, centres or institutes.

The full course would thus take a minimal time of approximately ten years. Procedure from stage to stage would depend on the necessary standard of competence being attained. Those who completed the course satisfactorily could be given an appropriate degree, such as Master of Surgery, Master of Medical Science or Master of Medicine. No further degrees would be conferred by the Faculty of Medicine, but those members with the necessary desire and special ability would be selected as consultants, directors or teachers, or to carry out special work. Subsequent training and teaching would consist of special lectures and demonstrations to ensure that every member was keeping abreast of recent advances in knowledge and technique.

Objections.

Finally, a few remarks about the objections usually advanced by those who oppose a national health service. It will be found, when one makes an honest effort and becomes informed of the true state of affairs, that the alleged objections are almost wholly invalid.

The statement that medical progress is dependent on the stimulus of competitive private practice is not true. It is, moreover, a gratuitous insult to the army of scientific workers who willingly spend their lives in an unremitting search for knowledge for a salary that is far too often inadequate. The implication that doctors need the spur of financial or other reward to make and keep them fully efficient should make every member of the profession feel ashamed.

The Australian Army Medical Corps, which is regimented to a high degree, is a salaried service. It is also a service in which there is almost a complete absence of choice of doctor by the patient and of patient by the doctor. Yet it would be absurd to suggest that the health of the army was not very well maintained or that members of the Australian Army Medical Corps tended to lose initiative, enterprise or efficiency.

Whether in a national service in peace-time there will be detrimental political interference or obnoxious bureaucratic control depends entirely on the profession. If the members cooperate intelligently in the setting up of an adequate, available service, they will determine control of it.

How the service is to be financed is a matter for the Government, and it is right that the money should come from the whole community. But whether it is collected as part of general taxation or in some other way is no concern of the profession. It is the profession's concern, however, to see that the poor are not further impoverished.

While the cost of such a service as has been outlined may be high, it would not be long before the expense was manifestly justified. With the institution of a better social system and a general knowledge of dietetics, the vitamin deficiency group of diseases would practically vanish. With better education, assured work and physiological fulfilment, psychiatric cases would decrease enormously. The study and practice of other aspects of prevention would rapidly decrease the number of other illnesses and disabilities.

Actually, in the scheme outlined in this article, there would be a minimum of regimentation, while there would be almost as great a choice of doctor and patient as there is at present. The only valid objection is that the doctor would be limited to a salary instead of being free to try to make a large income from his patients.

Conclusion.

A concerted, whole-hearted effort by the medical profession, primarily, and by the politicians and the people could rapidly give to Australia a national health service which would be an example to, and the envy of, the rest of the world.

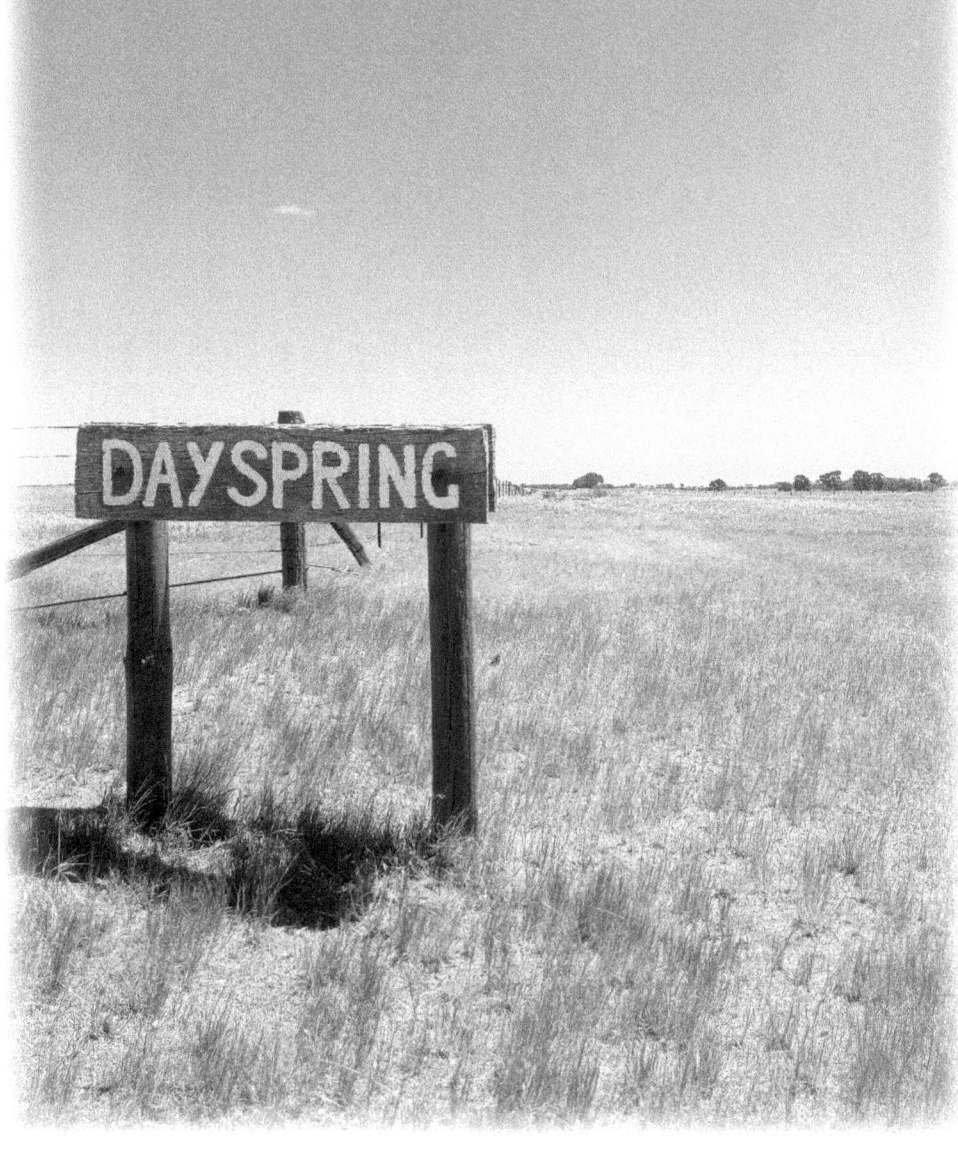

Wakefield Press is an independent publishing and
distribution company based in Adelaide, South Australia.
We love good stories and publish beautiful books.
To see our full range of books, please visit our website at
www.wakefieldpress.com.au
where all titles are available for purchase.
To keep up with our latest releases and news,
subscribe to the Wakefield Weekly at
https://mailchi.mp/wakefieldpress/subscribe

Find us!

Facebook: www.facebook.com/wakefield.press
Instagram: www.instagram.com/wakefieldpress

www.ingramcontent.com/pod-product-compliance
Lightning Source LLC
Chambersburg PA
CBHW040318170426
43197CB00021B/2955